THE DEMENTIA CARE TOOLKIT

Real Help for Challenging Behaviors and Caregiving Overwhelm

NATALI N. EDMONDS, PsyD, ABPP

JOSSEY-BASS™
A Wiley Brand

Published by John Wiley & Sons, Inc., Hoboken, New Jersey.

Library of Congress Cataloging-in-Publication Data is Available:

ISBN 9781394389636 (Paperback)
ISBN 9781394389650 (ePDF)
ISBN 9781394389643 (ePub)

Cover Design: Wiley
Cover Image: AlexeyVS/Getty Images
Author Photo: Sarah Hoag Photography

SKY10167734_090426

Praise for *The Dementia Care Toolkit*

"Most people become dementia caregivers with zero training—suddenly making decisions on the fly, unsure if they're getting anything right. Drawing on years of clinical experience, Natali Edmonds helps you move past the guesswork and into real solutions, giving you the tools to know exactly what to do instead of just hoping you're doing it right."

—Emma Heming Willis
caregiver advocate and *New York Times* best-selling author

"This masterful guide is an absolute lifeline for anyone navigating the profound complexities of Alzheimer's caregiving. By bridging the gap between clinical knowledge and daily reality, it delivers a transformative toolkit packed with actionable strategies for managing difficult behaviors. Dr. Edmonds arms care partners with knowledge and practical solutions aimed at improving their loved one's comfort and quality of life, reducing triggers for behaviors and distress, while also helping care partners to reduce their own stress. It is an essential and empowering guide for those navigating the challenging journey of cognitive impairment."

—Anna D. Burke, MD
Karsten Solheim for Dementia Research Chair, Medical Director of the Alzheimer's and Memory Disorders Program, Director of Neuropsychiatry, and Professor of Neurology at Barrow Neurological Institute

"I wish this book were handed to every single dementia caregiver the moment they stepped into this role. Dr. Natali is a gift to the dementia community."

—Carrie Aalberts
Dementia Darling

THE DEMENTIA CARE TOOLKIT

For dementia caregivers everywhere.

Those who show up day after day,

even when it hurts,

even when no one sees.

Contents

Preface

Caregiving is hard and heartbreaking. But you don't have to go through it alone.

We'll take this one step at a time.

Before we get into the challenges of dementia care and how to work through them, I want to introduce myself and share who this book is for.

My name is Natali Edmonds. I'm a board-certified geropsychologist. That means I'm a clinical psychologist trained in how aging, memory loss, and caregiving affect the brain, emotions, and daily life.

We're often called in when

- Caregivers need help responding to "behaviors" like aggression, wandering, or resistance.
- Families want testing to understand if memory or personality changes are dementia, normal aging, or something else.
- There's emotional overwhelm like grief, depression, anxiety, or a need to adjust to the difficult changes that come in later life.

In short, we focus on how the brain, emotions, and relationships shift with age, especially when dementia is involved.

Over the years, I've worked in memory care centers, home-based care programs, and hospital clinics. I've done cognitive testing, emotional counseling, and behavior consults. And while I valued that work, something always felt missing.

Too often, I met family members who were exhausted, overwhelmed, and desperate for answers, yet were given 30 minutes, a few brochures, and a follow-up appointment months away. That didn't sit right with me.

The healthcare system decided how much time I could spend with families and how many people I could see each day. So one day, in a moment of courage, I did something I had thought about for years but had always been too afraid to try. I turned on my camera and started sharing the kinds of conversations I'd been having with caregivers all along.

At night and on weekends, after seeing patients at the hospital or in their homes, I recorded videos sharing practical insights any family caregiver could start using right away. Those early videos eventually became the foundation of what is now the number one dementia training channel on YouTube.

From that work, Dementia Careblazers was born.

The word *Careblazer* is one I created. It describes caregivers who are looking for a new way forward, one that recognizes meaningful dementia support is needed beyond scheduled appointments and exam rooms.

If you picked up this book, you're already a Careblazer:

You're looking for better answers.

You're choosing not to settle.

You're open to doing things differently.

Dementia Careblazers didn't just serve the families I was seeing in hospitals and clinics. It became deeply personal as my own parents began showing signs of dementia. My personal caregiving experience isn't what led me into this field, but it profoundly shaped my understanding of it.

Because there's a big difference between learning about dementia and living it.

My education and credentials couldn't protect me from heartbreak, guilt, or mistakes. I've experienced all of them. And those experiences have made me even more committed to making sure the tools I share actually work in real life, not just in theory.

That's my promise to you in this book.

Everything I share comes from years of clinical experience and real-life caregiving moments, both my own and those of the thousands of caregivers I've worked with. Every tool you'll find here has been used, tested, and adapted in real homes by real families facing challenges very similar to yours.

Important note: Years ago, I interviewed a physician for my YouTube channel. He said caregivers should drink at least eight glasses of water a day. Simple enough, right?

Not for one viewer. He had a heart condition and was on fluid restrictions. Even five glasses of water could have been dangerous for him. Thankfully, he asked his doctor first, but he also emailed me to say he could never trust my videos again.

That experience reminded me that even the most common advice does not apply to everyone. That is why I want to be clear with you. This book is for educational purposes only. Even though I am a geropsychologist, I am not working as your or your loved one's healthcare provider. Nothing in these pages replaces the care you or your loved one receives from your medical team. My hope is that the tools and strategies here add to the care you already have.

Caregiving and dementia are never one-size-fits-all. What helps one person may not be right for another. Please use this book as a guide, not a prescription, and always check with your doctor or healthcare team if you are unsure.

Introduction

I'm sorry this book is in your hands right now, because it means someone in your life has dementia.

Your life as you once imagined it may feel like a distant memory, replaced by the constant needs of someone in your care.

Chances are you've already lived through some of the hardest parts of dementia caregiving, or you're bracing yourself for what might come next.

You may recognize some of these experiences:

- Not knowing what to say or what to do next
- The person with dementia not wanting your help
- The loneliness that comes as friends slowly disappear over years of caregiving
- The sadness of feeling like your yesterdays are brighter than your tomorrows
- The fear of not knowing whether your own health will last as long as your loved one needs you
- The anger toward family members who aren't helping

And unfortunately, the list goes on.

Dementia can make the people we've known most of our lives feel like strangers.

It can make the comfort of our own homes feel more like hospital rooms.

It can make us feel like we are never doing enough, even when we are giving everything we have.

I could fill these pages with the challenges dementia caregiving brings.

I'm guessing you could, too.

But I don't want this book to focus only on what's hard.

I want it to focus on what can help.

My Goal with This Book

We may not be able to cure the disease yet, but there *are* things we can do to make this easier.

While this book focuses on how to respond to loved ones with dementia when they are showing confusing or challenging behaviors, it also focuses on how to reduce the emotional harm caregiving can do to you in the process.

This is not a book on how to be better.

It is a book on how to suffer less while doing something impossibly hard.

The fact that you're reading this tells me you're trying. For many caregivers, the hardest part isn't what they're doing. It's watching things get worse anyway.

Easier doesn't always mean calmer days or fewer symptoms. Often, it means less self-blame, less escalation, and less second-guessing how you handled things.

That's my goal for this book.

To share tools that have helped thousands of other caregivers find relief, steadiness, and sometimes even moments of joy along this confusing and heartbreaking journey.

I'll share practical, creative, and often simple approaches drawn from years of working with caregivers like you. The stories throughout this book are real, though names and identifying details have been changed.

I'm sorry this is the book you need. But I'm grateful you found it, and I hope it helps you more than you expect.

What This Book Is and Is Not

This is not a medical textbook. You won't find long disease descriptions or complicated charts. You'll find practical tools and clear explanations to help you understand what's happening and what you can do to make daily life easier for both you and the person you're caring for.

This book is for family caregivers who need real solutions without having to wait months for another rushed appointment.

I will never pretend to have all the answers. But I do want to share what I know, what I've learned, and what has helped many caregivers like you. While you may not use every tool in this book, I'm confident you'll find some that make a meaningful difference.

How to Use This Book

Now that you know why I wrote this book, let's move to the part that matters most: helping you feel more supported and less overwhelmed.

In the pages ahead, you'll learn why behaviors happen, how to respond in ways that don't make things worse, and how to protect your own health in the process. You'll find ideas for the person you're caring for and for yourself.

This book is divided into three parts. Each one serves a different purpose. Together, they are meant to help you understand what is happening and how you can respond.

Part I: The Foundation: Understanding Dementia Behaviors and Yourself: The first part is about understanding what is happening.

Not just in your loved one's brain, but in the moments that leave you confused, frustrated, or questioning yourself. We look at why certain behaviors show up, why they can feel so personal, and why even when you are trying your best, things can still unravel.

These chapters help the tools in the rest of the book work better.

Part II: The Strategies: Focusing on the Person with Dementia: The second part is practical. It's filled with strategies that have worked for real caregivers in real homes, not just in textbooks or training manuals.

Return to this section whenever a new behavior appears or an old one shifts. You don't need to memorize every strategy or use them all. But you will likely find a few that make difficult moments easier to manage.

Use what fits your current situation. Then come back when things change.

Part III: The Support: Focusing on the Caregiver: Caregivers are already doing everything they can just to get through the day. Being told to "take care of yourself" can feel frustrating. It sounds nice, but it doesn't tell you how to actually do that while you're caregiving.

This third and final part is about helping you manage the heartbreak and emotional toll that comes with caregiving. This is not about bubble baths or adding more to your already full plate. It's about protecting your energy and your ability to keep going in a role that can last years, sometimes decades.

Return to this section when doubt, anger, resentment, or guilt start to build. It's here to support you, not to give you more to do.

You don't need to read this book straight through. You don't need to read it in order. And you don't need to use everything in it. You are welcome to skip around and focus on the chapters that speak most to what you're dealing with right now. I hope you'll keep this book nearby and return to it when you need support or reassurance that you're not alone.

If at any point this book feels like too much, it's okay to put it down and come back later. Support should reduce pressure, not add to it. The book will be waiting for you when you're ready to pick it back up again.

I've created some free companion resources to help you apply what you're learning in real life. You can find those at www.careblazers.com/book.

Part I

The Foundation: Understanding Dementia Behaviors and Yourself

Chapter 1

Understanding Dementia

Dementia is one of the most misunderstood conditions, even by well-meaning professionals.

If you've found yourself confused by what you're seeing with your loved one, there's a reason for that. Dementia doesn't affect every brain the same way, and it doesn't progress in a predictable, straight line. What you're noticing may not match what you expected, what others describe, or what you've seen in movies.

This chapter will help you understand what dementia is and is not so you can stop questioning yourself. We'll start by going over the difference between dementia and Alzheimer's disease.

Alzheimer's Disease Versus Dementia

Sometimes dementia and Alzheimer's are talked about as if they mean the same thing. Other times, people talk as if they are completely different. All of this adds to the confusion many caregivers already feel.

Here's the simplest way to think about it: *dementia* is a general term. It describes ongoing problems with thinking, memory, and daily functioning caused by changes in the brain. It is not a specific diagnosis on its own.

Alzheimer's disease is the most common cause of dementia, but it's not the only one. Other causes include Lewy body dementia, frontotemporal dementia, and vascular dementia, among others.

In simple terms, dementia is a category, not a single diagnosis.

A helpful comparison is the word *cancer*. Cancer is a category, not a specific diagnosis. In the same way there are many types of cancer, there are many types of dementia.

When someone is told they have dementia due to Alzheimer's disease, it means that Alzheimer's is the disease causing the dementia symptoms you're seeing. But when someone is told they have dementia, it doesn't necessarily tell you which disease is causing it. Many caregivers are told their loved one "has dementia," but no one explains what kind or whether it matters.

No matter the type, all dementias affect thinking in ways that eventually interfere with a person's ability to live safely on their own day-to-day. This often shows up as difficulty managing finances, driving safely, cooking meals, keeping track of medications, or living alone.

For many families, it begins with small moments that are easy to brush off at first. A pot left on the stove. A medication taken twice. A door left unlocked. Looking back, many caregivers realize these were early signs that the brain was struggling to do things it once handled automatically.

Eventually, all forms of dementia reach a point where additional support is needed to stay safe. That support most often comes from family caregivers.

Not knowing the specific type doesn't mean you missed something or failed to advocate. It's actually extremely common not to know.

I meet new caregivers every week, and most do not know what type of dementia their loved one has. Many do not even have an official diagnosis. Some were never directly told at all. Some discover dementia is part of the picture only after reading medical records, sometimes months or years later.

My own parents never received a formal diagnosis of a specific type of dementia.

While understanding different dementia types can be helpful, not everyone gets clear answers. Some people have more than one type at the same time, known as *mixed dementia*. In other cases, providers are unable to determine the exact cause, which is often documented as *unspecified dementia*.

Sometimes the picture becomes clearer over time as new symptoms appear. Other times, it never does. That uncertainty is far more common than most caregivers realize.

What matters most right now is not having a perfect label. What matters is understanding how dementia affects thinking and daily life so you can respond with more confidence.

Dementia Is Not a Normal Part of Aging

Age is the biggest risk factor for dementia, but dementia itself is not a normal part of aging.

Just as our chances of getting in a car accident increase the more time we spend on the road, our chances of developing dementia increase the longer we live.

Some thinking changes are normal as we get older, such as needing more time to think things through or having trouble finding the right words. These changes don't automatically make it difficult for us to take care of ourselves.

When thinking changes begin to interfere with safety, judgment, or everyday functioning, that is when it's no longer considered normal aging.

This difference matters. Many caregivers are told, or come to believe, that what they are seeing is "just age." Understanding that dementia is not a normal part of aging helps caregivers trust their observations, seek help sooner, and advocate more confidently.

If all of this feels confusing, it's not because you're missing something. Dementia is complicated, and it doesn't always make sense.

"Is There a Point in Getting a Diagnosis?"

Many families wonder whether formal testing is worth it, especially when there is no cure. A full evaluation can be time-consuming and emotionally exhausting, and some caregivers are told there is no real point in testing.

One important reason families consider an evaluation is that some conditions can look very much like dementia but are actually treatable. I often call these *dementia look-alikes.*

For example, depression in older adults can mimic dementia. Someone may withdraw, lose motivation, struggle with concentration, or stop keeping up with daily care. Without an evaluation, these changes can be mistaken for dementia when they may improve with the right treatment.

Other issues that can look like dementia include untreated hearing loss, medication side effects, nutritional deficiencies, thyroid problems, dehydration, or sleep disorders. Identifying these doesn't rule out dementia, but it can still improve thinking and daily functioning in meaningful ways.

Another reason families pursue evaluation is for understanding and peace of mind. While no one wants to hear that someone they love has dementia, many caregivers describe a sense of relief knowing there is an explanation for what they've been seeing. A diagnosis can help families stop questioning themselves and begin planning for the future with clearer expectations.

In some cases, early assessment may also open the door to treatment options or support services that require documentation.

Whether or not to pursue testing is a personal decision. What matters most is understanding why evaluation can be helpful, so you can decide what feels right for you and your family.

"It Can't Be Dementia; Her Memory Is Fine"

When most people think about dementia, they think about memory loss. That makes sense, because memory problems are the main symptom in Alzheimer's disease.

But memory loss is not always required.

Some dementias affect behavior, personality, judgment, language, or problem-solving first. Memory may appear okay, especially early on.

Thinking abilities include more than memory. They include attention, judgment, language, social awareness, and coordination. A significant decline in even one of these areas can interfere with safety and independence.

This is why dementia can look very different from person to person.

Dementia doesn't have a single look or pattern.

Comparing your experience to someone else's often creates unnecessary fear. Hearing another caregiver's story does not mean that is what is coming next for your loved one.

In early stages, many people with dementia remain active in their communities. They may still drive, live alone, work, volunteer, or manage daily responsibilities.

This can make caregiving especially isolating. Others may only see brief snapshots where your loved one seems fine, while you live the full picture day after day. When others don't see what you see, caregivers can be left feeling like they are exaggerating or overreacting, even when they are not.

Over time, abilities change. Risks increase. More supervision becomes necessary.

It is not the diagnosis that takes away freedoms. It is how the disease affects current abilities.

"They Did Just Fine Yesterday"

One of the most confusing parts of dementia is that ability is not lost all at once.

In early stages especially, dementia affects consistency before it affects ability.

A person may manage a task one day and struggle with the same task the next. They may seem clear in the morning and confused later that same afternoon.

This inconsistency causes many caregivers to second-guess what they're seeing. Are they pretending? Is this really dementia?

Dementia does not progress in a straight line. Skills can come and go, even as overall decline continues. A good day does not mean the dementia is gone. A difficult day does not mean everything has suddenly changed.

Both can exist at the same time.

It's easy to overlook symptoms early on. Many people are already in the moderate stages of dementia by the time they have their first formal evaluation, often because changes happened slowly and gradually.

This is not something to be upset with yourself about.

Just as it's hard to notice our own aging when we look in the mirror every day, it's hard to see slow changes in someone we love and see regularly.

A friend of mine has a mother who was diagnosed with early-onset Alzheimer's disease, meaning symptoms began before age 65. Her parents were physically strong and active, and they trained together for a half marathon in Arizona.

On the day of the race, her dad finished first and waited at the finish line. As time passed and she never arrived, panic set in. Based on her training, she should have finished long ago.

Eventually, they found her. She was safe, but she had become lost on the trails.

That day, the family realized that ability did not equal safety.

This back-and-forth is often harder to adjust to than steady decline. It keeps many caregivers in a constant state of emotional tension and self-doubt.

Key Takeaways

- Dementia is a category, not a single diagnosis. Alzheimer's disease is one cause, but there are many others.
- Not knowing the exact type does not mean you missed something or failed to advocate. Unfortunately, uncertainty is common.
- Dementia is not a normal part of aging. When thinking changes begin to interfere with safety and daily life, that is different from typical age-related changes.
- Memory loss is not always the first or main symptom. Changes in judgment, behavior, language, or personality can appear first.

- Dementia does not progress in a straight line. Good days and difficult days can exist at the same time.
- Ability does not always equal safety. A person may still be capable of doing something and no longer be safe doing it.
- Confusion about what you are seeing is not a sign that you are doing something wrong. Dementia itself is complex and inconsistent.

Looking Ahead

Dementia is complex, unpredictable, and deeply misunderstood.

If you've felt confused about dementia, testing, or the symptoms you're seeing, that's a natural response to something that can change over time and look very different from one person to another.

You don't need perfect answers or timelines to keep moving forward.

As dementia changes the brain, it changes how your loved one understands what's happening, communicates, and responds. What you see on the outside often shows up as behaviors.

In Chapter 2, you'll learn why those behaviors happen and how understanding what drives them can reduce stress, burnout, and difficult decisions about safety and care.

Chapter 2

Why People with Dementia Display "Difficult" Behaviors

We were sitting in a virtual support room—about 20 Careblazers who gather week after week to share tears, breakthroughs, and everything in between.

The group started like it always does. Someone was sharing a recent caregiving moment. Then, without warning, we heard a man's voice yelling through one participant's unmuted computer.

"Stop lying, you stupid b*@!h!" The room went silent. Her husband was yelling at the top of his lungs. Accusing her. Calling her names.

This wasn't a bad relationship.

This wasn't a caregiving mistake.

This was dementia.

This is how dementia can look. It's unsettling. It's painful. And for many caregivers, it's completely unexpected. It's a reality many caregivers are living every day. Dementia can be cruel. It can turn homes into tense, unpredictable places. And it can leave caregivers questioning everything they're doing.

If you've been caring for someone with dementia for any length of time, chances are you've already seen behaviors like yelling, pacing, accusing, refusing care, resisting help, or even physical aggression. Or you may be seeing the opposite, like your loved one pulling back, doing less, or losing interest in things they used to enjoy.

Moments like these are often the most distressing part of caregiving, especially when your efforts to help are met with anger, suspicion, or rejection. It can feel like nothing you do is right. Like your loved one is angry at you, even though all you are trying to do is help.

What matters most for you right now is this: **these behaviors aren't random and they aren't personal, even though it often feels that way.**

Even when we understand why dementia-related behaviors happen, that understanding doesn't make responding to them easy. Knowing these common causes won't magically erase the exhaustion, frustration, or heartbreak that comes with facing them day after day.

These behaviors can feel confusing and personal. But they don't come out of nowhere, even when they seem to. There's usually something driving them under the surface.

The best chance of changing a difficult dementia-related behavior is to start by trying to understand it. And we can't do that if we're only focused on stopping the behavior.

Let's start with one of the most common and misunderstood reasons.

Reason 1: Lack of Awareness: "Tell Him He Has Dementia!"

I can still picture her sitting across from me in my office.

Her shoulders were tense. Her face was tired. Her voice carried a quiet desperation.

"Please," she said. "Tell him he has dementia."

A few months earlier, I had tested her husband. The results were clear. He had dementia, likely of the Alzheimer's type, already in the moderate stage.

Like many caregivers, she had noticed changes long before the diagnosis. The testing only confirmed what she already feared. Still, hearing it out loud made everything feel final. Real.

Now she was back, pleading with me to tell him again.

Of course, I already had. Just months earlier, a full medical team had sat with them, explained the diagnosis, written it down, and shared recommendations and resources.

And yet, here she was, asking me to repeat it.

I knew what she was hoping for.

So I asked, "Tell me what you're hoping will happen if I tell him again."

She didn't hesitate.

"He'll stop resisting my help," she said. "He still thinks he can do everything on his own."

She went on to explain that he didn't believe anything was wrong. She reminded him of the diagnosis. She explained it again and again. Nothing changed.

What she was facing is one of the most common and painful challenges in dementia caregiving. It's when the person with dementia doesn't believe anything is wrong with them.

> They may not believe they have dementia.
>
> They may believe they can still do everything they've always done. To caregivers, this looks like denial. But it isn't. This symptom has a name. It's called *anosognosia*.

Anosognosia is a neurological loss of awareness. The brain is no longer able to recognize its own changes. It is not stubbornness. It is not refusal. And it is not something the person is choosing.

Unlike denial, which is an emotional response to painful information, anosognosia is neurological. It happens when the parts of the brain responsible for insight are affected.

Insight is the ability to understand that something is wrong and how it affects you. Dementia commonly damages the brain regions that support this ability.

That means many people with dementia genuinely cannot understand what you understand.

And because this loss of awareness is brain-based, no amount of explaining, reminding, or reasoning can restore it.

Simply put, there is nothing we can say or do that will make them see what their brain can no longer process.

This helps explain why resistance to help can feel so intense.

From their perspective, help may feel unnecessary, intrusive, or even threatening. Most of us would deeply resist personal help if we didn't believe we needed it.

Trying to convince someone with anosognosia that they need help is like trying to get a blind person to see by asking them to look harder. No amount of effort will change what the brain can no longer do.

Anosognosia isn't just frustrating. It can be dangerous.

When someone is unaware of their limitations, they may insist on activities that put them at risk. For example:

- Driving a car or taking public transport
- Using tools or appliances
- Managing medications

I once worked with a Careblazer whose husband believed he could still safely do electrical work around the house. She walked in one day to find him working with live wires.

Another man I evaluated was referred after driving his car into the front of a building. He had confused the gas and brake pedals and insisted he was still safe to drive.

Thankfully, no one was injured in either case.

When anosognosia is present, caregiver burden is often higher. The responsibility of keeping someone safe while they insist they don't need help is heavy.

We'll talk throughout this book about how to approach safety with dignity and care. For now, what matters most is this: anosognosia is real.

And one of the most damaging things we can do is repeatedly try to convince someone they need help or remind them of their diagnosis. That approach usually increases distress, escalates resistance, and strains the relationship.

This isn't about you. It's about changes in the brain.

Some important points to remember:

- Anosognosia is a loss of awareness caused by brain changes, not denial.
- The person is not being stubborn or difficult on purpose.
- You cannot convince someone of something their brain is no longer able to understand.

Reason 2: The Relationship: "He's Nice to Everyone Except Me"

I remember how much it used to bother me that everyone who met my dad seemed to love him right away.

They'd say things like:

"He's so fun."

"He's such a great guy."

"He's so nice."

You'd think I'd be happy to hear that. But the truth is, it got under my skin.

I didn't get to see that side of him very much anymore.

As my dad became more ill, I started to see a different version of him—demanding, irritable, sometimes condescending. It felt like no matter what I did, it was never enough, even though I was the one doing the things that mattered most.

I took him to appointments.

Made sure he had food.

Changed the dressings on his wounds.

I was giving so much. And yet, it felt like he resented me.

The people who stopped by for a short visit or called on the phone seemed to get the best version of him.

Me, the one there day after day, seemed to get the worst of it. I'm not proud to admit that. But it's true.

One afternoon, I was sitting next to him while he watched the same news program on repeat. And that's when something clicked.

Our entire relationship had become about caregiving.

Somewhere along the way, I stopped being his daughter and became his nurse, his assistant, his protector. This happened quietly, gradually, and not on purpose.

In our effort to be good caregivers, we become the person who brings limits, reminders, schedules, and corrections. The person who steps in when something isn't safe. The person who represents what has been lost.

We mean well. We're trying to help. We're trying to keep them safe.

But to the person with dementia, that constant presence can begin to feel uncomfortable, restrictive, or threatening, even if they can't explain why.

When the relationship shifts, behaviors start to shift with it.

Even when someone with dementia forgets what you said or did, their brain often remembers how they felt.

This is called *emotional memory.*

Emotional memory allows feelings to stick, even when details fade. Over time, those feelings shape how someone responds to you, even if they don't know why.

This helps explain a painful pattern many caregivers recognize:

Why your loved one may be pleasant with visitors but resistant with you.

Why short interactions go smoothly, while longer ones feel tense.

Why the person doing the most gets the most pushback.

This doesn't mean you've done something wrong.

It often means you're the one who's there.

Your loved one may not remember that you smiled earlier. They may not understand that your stressed expression has nothing to do with them. But they can still remember how it feels when you're around. And over time, those feelings can start to shape how they respond.

Caregivers often describe feeling like the "bad guy," the "warden," or the "boss." They wonder why their loved one seems kinder to everyone else.

This is one of the most painful parts of dementia caregiving. Not because you're doing something wrong.

But because dementia changes how the relationship is experienced.

When the relationship feels strained, behaviors often follow.

This also explains why repeatedly forcing a loved one to do something they strongly resist can make future cooperation less likely. Each tense interaction strengthens the emotional memory tied to the relationship.

This doesn't mean the relationship is broken beyond repair.

It means the disease is influencing how connection is felt.

Understanding this doesn't erase the hurt. But it does help explain why behaviors often show up most intensely with the person doing the most.

Some important points to remember:

- Dementia can strain relationships even when love and effort are present.
- The person doing the most caregiving often receives the most resistance.
- Emotional memory allows feelings to persist even when details are forgotten.

Reason 3: Resentment over Loss of Control: "Everything Is Being Decided for Her Now"

Imagine if someone else decided what you'd eat, when you'd sleep, what you'd wear, and whether or not you could leave the house. Every. Single. Day.

Even if they meant well. Even if they loved you deeply. Wouldn't some part of you want to push back?

For many people with dementia, this slow and steady loss of control is one of the most distressing parts of the disease. And it often shows up as behaviors caregivers find confusing, illogical, or flat-out defiant.

One Careblazer described it perfectly when she wrote, "It's like everything is being decided for her now, and she's fighting back in the only way she knows how—by saying no."

Sometimes, people with dementia resist care even when the relationship itself is strong.

As the disease progresses, independence slips away in layers. What starts as needing help with driving or managing finances can turn into no longer choosing what to eat, what to wear, or how to spend the day. Appointments are scheduled for them. Visitors arrive without warning. Daily routines fill up with plans made by others.

So when you cheerfully remind your loved one that their favorite TV show is about to start and they snap at you, it can feel like it came out of nowhere. But when so much of life is happening *to* them instead of *with* them, even the smallest prompt can feel like another loss of control.

When most things are being decided for them, a person with dementia may assert control in the one place they still can: their willingness. In those moments, the behavior is often less about what's being asked and more about the fact that someone else is deciding.

This isn't because you've done anything wrong. If anything, you're likely doing everything you can to make life easier and safer. But from their perspective, it can feel like being swept along in a life they didn't choose.

In psychology, this response is called *reactance*. It's a natural human drive to protect autonomy when it feels threatened. When people sense their freedom is being taken away, they often try to get it back by doing the opposite of what's being asked.

So when a family member says it's time for a shower and the person with dementia refuses, the resistance may not be about the shower itself. It may be about protecting the only thing they feel they have left: the power to say no.

At its core, this kind of resistance is often an attempt to say: *I still matter. My voice still matters.*

Understanding this doesn't make the behavior easy. But it does make it make sense.

Some important points to remember:

- Loss of control plays a major role in many dementia-related behaviors.
- Saying no is often an attempt to protect independence, not reject you.
- Resistance is frequently automatic, not intentional or manipulative.

Reason 4: Reacting to Unmet Needs: "I Just Thought She Was Being Stubborn"

People with dementia often struggle to meet needs most of us manage automatically. If they're cold, they may not think to grab a sweater. If they're hungry, they may not remember how to find food. If they're in pain, they may not be able to explain it. If they're overstimulated, they may not know how to make their environment calmer.

Pain, hunger, discomfort, fear, or the need to use the bathroom can all show up as behavior when a person with dementia can't recognize or communicate what's wrong. When this happens, the behavior isn't a sign they're being difficult. More often, it's a sign that something important isn't being met.

What makes this so difficult is that dementia gets in the way of a person realizing their own needs, remembering what to do about them, or putting those needs into words.

Imagine this: You're sitting in the living room and suddenly you feel thirsty. You'd probably get up and get a glass of water. Simple.

For a person with dementia, that same situation isn't simple at all.

They may not recognize that they're thirsty.

They may not remember how to get water.

They may not be able to explain what they want.

So instead of saying, "I'm thirsty," they might pace, yell, or become restless. They might try to leave the house, searching for something they can't name.

From the outside, the behavior can look random or confusing. From the inside, it often makes sense.

Meaningful Expressions

This is why many dementia-related behaviors are not meaningless. They are *expressions*. The person is trying to express something they need or want but no longer has the ability to explain directly.

Understandably, caregivers tend to focus on the behavior itself. They want it to stop. These behaviors are exhausting, disruptive, and sometimes frightening.

But when we focus only on stopping the behavior, we can miss what the behavior is trying to tell us.

Think again about the thirst example. If we stop the pacing but never offer water, the person is still thirsty.

Sometimes the unmet need is physical. Other times it's emotional or environmental. And sometimes it's about comfort or dignity, not safety.

For example, a person with dementia may resist showering not because they don't want to be clean, but because being naked feels embarrassing, cold, or vulnerable. They may not be able to explain that discomfort, so it shows up as refusal, agitation, or anger.

In situations like this, meeting the need can look surprisingly simple. Allowing them to wear boxers, underwear, or a light nightgown in the shower. Warming up the bathroom first. Covering them with a towel and uncovering only one area at a time.

When we focus only on the "problem behavior," we miss an opportunity to help. We're so focused on making the behavior stop that we never uncover what's causing it.

Here are some common unmet needs that can show up as behaviors:

- Physical discomfort such as pain, hunger, thirst, or fatigue
- Emotional distress such as fear, anxiety, or sadness
- Social needs such as loneliness, boredom, or lack of stimulation
- Environmental issues such as noise, clutter, or chaos
- Personal preferences such as privacy, favorite foods, or familiar routines

Many of these needs don't announce themselves clearly. They show up as clues.

Understanding Human Frustration

Think about a time when something small but familiar wasn't available. Your favorite snack is gone. A room feels uncomfortable. Someone else controls the TV. Even in those moments, irritation or restlessness can appear. The difference is that your brain can usually regulate the feeling. You can wait, reason with yourself, or adapt.

A person with dementia often can't.

It's important to pause here.

Understanding unmet needs doesn't mean you are expected to figure everything out.

Caregivers often feel overwhelmed by this idea, as if they are supposed to identify the exact right need every time. Hunger. Pain. Fear. Boredom. Temperature. Modesty. Fatigue. Loneliness. The list can feel endless.

And the truth is, you won't always know. Sometimes you will make a thoughtful guess and it won't help. Sometimes there will be multiple needs at once. And sometimes there will be no clear unmet need at all. What matters is that you're not just reacting to the behavior, but considering what might be behind it.

That said, it's important to be clear: **many dementia-related behaviors are driven by unmet needs or desires. But not all of them.**

Some behaviors happen even when needs are met, care is thoughtful, and the environment is supportive.

Those behaviors are the direct result of brain changes, which I talk about next.

Some important points to remember:

- Many behaviors are attempts to meet a need that can't be identified or expressed.
- Behavior often becomes communication when words and insight are lost.
- Not all behaviors come from unmet needs, but many do.

Reason 5: Brain Changes: "It Doesn't Matter How Calm or Kind I Am, He Still Yells at Me"

When caregivers hear tips about how to respond to dementia-related behaviors, it can sometimes feel like an unspoken message is being sent: if only you responded better, this wouldn't be happening.

You may have even heard that all behavior is communication and that if you can just uncover the message, you can solve the behavior.

While well-intentioned, this idea carries a quiet blame. It can leave you feeling like the only reason your loved one continues to have behaviors is because you have not yet figured out the right approach.

Put bluntly, it can feel like their behaviors are happening because you are not responding the "right" way.

That is exhausting. And it is not true.

The truth is, even the most loving, patient, and skilled caregiver can face difficult behaviors. Not because they are failing, but because dementia changes the brain in ways no amount of caregiving can undo.

Not every behavior is meant to communicate something.

And not every behavior is something you can figure out or prevent.

Sometimes, a behavior is simply the result of brain changes.

Here is one of the most important principles to understand: anything that affects the brain will affect behavior. The brain controls how we reason, communicate, regulate emotions, and respond to the world. When the brain changes, behavior changes.

Think of the brain like a computer. On the outside, it may look the same. But when something inside the system starts to fail, the computer does not work the way it used to. It freezes. It misfires. It produces errors.

Dementia does the same thing to the brain. With dementia, brain cells die. The brain physically shrinks. Blood flow is reduced.

Communication between brain regions slows or breaks down. Tasks that once required little effort become overwhelming or impossible.

You can't see this damage directly. But you can see the result in the behaviors, the confusion, and the reactions that don't always make sense to you. But they *do* make sense given what the brain can no longer do.

These invisible changes are one reason caregivers often wonder if the person is pretending or being manipulative. After all, how can someone seem fine one moment and completely confused the next?

But the brain is changing moment by moment.

Trying harder, doing more, or being "better" at caregiving cannot reverse dying brain cells.

No matter how thoughtful or skilled you are, there will be behaviors that still happen. And that is not a failure.

There are brain networks involved in how we experience reality. In some cases, especially those with Alzheimer's disease, brain scans can identify changes in these brain networks that predict who will experience hallucinations or delusions before they ever appear.

That means when those networks are affected, no amount of reassurance, logic, or caregiving skill can fully prevent the symptoms that follow.

Simply put, some behaviors are biologically driven from the start. They are not caused by poor caregiving. There is no unmet need or desire to figure out. They are caused by the disease.

This does not mean we stop supporting our loved ones or trying to improve quality of life. But it does mean we stop blaming ourselves when things do not go perfectly.

Sometimes it is not about your approach. It is about what the brain can no longer do.

At the same time, we do not want to assume every behavior is caused only by brain changes. If we do, we risk missing things we actually can address, such as pain, fear, boredom, or unmet needs. Both can be true.

There is always something we can do to support our loved one, even when we can't stop a behavior entirely.

Some important points to remember:

- Not all behavior is communication. Some are caused by changes in the brain.
- Not all behaviors are something to be solved or figured out.
- It's okay to talk with your loved one's healthcare provider about medication options, especially if the behavior is causing lots of distress for your loved one.

Considering Medication

This is also when medication may come into the picture. It's not usually the first place to start for dementia-related behaviors, but it can be helpful in situations where distress is high or safety is a concern.

I once spoke with a Careblazer whose mother woke every night screaming in terror because she believed she was being attacked. The daughter tried everything: comfort, reassurance, redirection. Nothing helped.

When considering medication, the question is not, "Does this behavior bother me?"

It is, "Is this distressing for them?"

Her mother lived in fear every night.

In situations like this, medication is not about making caregiving easier. It is about reducing suffering.

If a person is experiencing ongoing emotional or physical distress, or if behaviors put them or others at risk, talk with their healthcare provider about whether medication might help. The goal is relief, not sedation. Comfort, not control.

Even then, medication is never the whole answer. It does not replace supportive responses. It may take the edge off, but it does not eliminate the need for compassion and understanding.

Understanding that some behaviors are the direct result of brain changes helps you to let go of guilt and focus on what is within your control: how you respond.

Key Takeaways

- Many behaviors are not intentional or manipulative. They are the result of how dementia is affecting the brain's ability to process information, regulate emotions, and make sense of the world.
- You don't need to identify the exact cause every time. Even considering these possibilities can help you approach difficult moments with more clarity and less resentment.
- When a behavior appears, try asking yourself, "What might be driving this?" That shift can lead to calmer and more effective responses.

Looking Ahead

It's one thing to understand possible reasons for the behaviors we are seeing. It's another to know what to actually do when they happen.

In Part II, I share dozens of caregiving tools you can use for all kinds of different behaviors, regardless of the underlying cause. But those tools won't be as helpful if you are already overwhelmed, depleted, or running on empty.

While most dementia resources focus almost exclusively on how to help the person with dementia feel calmer or safer, it's very important to understand what this experience does to the caregiver. If we truly want to improve life for people living with dementia, we must also support the people caring for them.

That is where we go next.

In Chapter 3, we will shift the focus to you. We will talk about the emotional weight of dementia caregiving and what can help make this journey feel more manageable, even when it remains undeniably hard. Because caring well for someone with dementia starts with caring well for the caregiver.

That is you.

When you're ready, turn the page.

Chapter 3

Why You Don't Actually Want to Feel Better All the Time (and What to Do Instead)

By simply being alive, we are going to experience emotional pain.

Life is not gentle all the time. It comes with loss, disappointment, heartbreak, and moments that change us forever. As long as we are living, loving, and caring about anything at all, pain will be part of the experience.

That has always been true for you.

Long before dementia entered your life, you've faced hard things.

A relationship that did not turn out the way you hoped.

A job or opportunity that slipped away.

A loss you never fully recovered from.

A moment when life clearly did not go according to plan.

No one gets through life without pain.

Right now, caregiving happens to be one of the painful chapters you are living through.

And here is something that is not said often enough: caregiving will still hurt sometimes.

No matter how many books you read.

No matter how many support groups you attend.

No matter how skilled, loving, or informed you become.

That doesn't mean you are doing it wrong.

It means you are human.

It's unlikely that this episode of your life will be one of the happiest. There may be moments of joy in caregiving, but there are also moments of deep heartbreak. Measuring each phase by how happy you feel will often leave you discouraged.

Instead of asking how happy you are, it may be more helpful to ask how meaningful this season of your life is.

You are giving your time, energy, attention, and often your own resources to keep another person safe when they can no longer do that for themselves.

That may not make this season joyful. But it does make it meaningful.

And since emotional pain has always been a part of being human, maybe the goal isn't to avoid pain altogether. Maybe the real goal is learning how to carry it without it breaking us.

That's what this chapter is about.

The Problem with Trying to Feel Good All the Time

Many caregivers carry quiet beliefs like these:

"I'm not supposed to feel this bad."

"I should be coping better."

"Nothing I do is right."

But what if those beliefs are actually making things harder?

When you believe you should feel okay all the time, every hard emotion starts to feel like something you need to fix. But if you're honest, there are many things in this world you probably don't *want* to feel good about.

War.

Suffering.

Injustice.

Or the fact that someone we love has dementia.

Feeling bad about those things makes sense.

So if you wouldn't want to feel good about life's hardest realities, then it follows that you aren't meant to feel good all the time.

One Careblazer said it simply during a support meeting: "Unfortunately, this is going to hurt."

That sentence holds a lot of wisdom.

Instead of putting all our energy into trying to feel better as fast as possible, what if we put more energy into learning how to handle the hurt when it shows up?

Feeling Bad Is Not the Problem

When caregivers first hear this idea, it can sound discouraging. Some think, "So I'm just going to feel awful forever?"

No. That is not what this means.

This is not about resigning yourself to misery.

And it's not about giving up on feeling better.

It's about stopping the fight against feelings that make sense.

Feeling sad about dementia doesn't mean something has gone wrong.

Feeling angry, overwhelmed, or filled with grief doesn't mean you are failing.

It means you are responding normally to something that is genuinely hard.

What actually makes things worse is

- Being upset about being upset
- Judging yourself for how you feel
- Believing you shouldn't feel this way

Feeling bad is not the problem.
Believing you should never feel bad is.

There are absolutely ways to feel lighter and more grounded. We'll talk about those soon. But before we talk about changing how you feel, it's important to make sure we aren't unintentionally adding more suffering by fighting emotions that make sense.

Caregiving often gets easier when we stop telling ourselves we're doing something wrong just because it hurts.

We spend a lot of time talking about how to feel better. But almost no one teaches us how to sit with the hurt.

Knowing how to sit with sadness, grief, anger, or fear is just as important as knowing how to feel calm or hopeful. This isn't about wallowing or giving up. It's about building trust in yourself.

Trust that you can feel something painful and still keep going.

Trust that emotions can rise without ruining you.

Trust that discomfort does not mean danger.

Emotional Waves

It can help to think about emotions like waves in the ocean.

Sometimes the water is calm. Other times the waves are rough and knock you off balance. The ocean isn't broken when the waves are strong. It's just being the ocean.

Emotions work the same way. They rise. They peak. They fall. No feeling stays exactly the same forever.

Instead of asking, "How do I make this stop?" a more helpful question is, "How do I want to respond when this hurts?" Because the pain itself may not be optional. But how you relate to it is.

This is where relief begins. And it's where we'll go next.

Yes, caregiving is going to hurt sometimes. That is not your fault. It's the reality of loving someone through a disease that keeps taking more as you keep giving more.

But here is the good news.

A lot of what makes caregiving feel unbearable is not only what's happening around you. It's what's happening inside you at the same time. The meaning you make. The pressure you put on yourself. The belief that you shouldn't feel this way.

Key Takeaways

- Emotional pain in caregiving is not a sign of failure. It's a healthy and human response to loving someone through something genuinely hard.
- Trying to feel good all the time often adds more suffering than the pain itself, especially when we judge or resist emotions that make sense.
- Relief isn't about making the hurt disappear. Sometimes it means learning how to live with it without turning against yourself.

Looking Ahead

This chapter isn't about learning to tolerate misery. It's about removing the extra suffering that comes from fighting emotions that make sense.

In Chapter 4, we'll begin talking about how your thoughts shape how hard emotions hit—and how to work with your mind in a way that actually helps.

You will still have hard moments.

But they won't knock you down in the same way.

When you're ready, turn the page.

Chapter 4

Your Ability to Change Feelings

This chapter will show you how to start feeling better.

But that doesn't mean you should always try to feel better.

Cognitive behavioral therapy (CBT) is a type of therapy psychologists use to help people who feel anxious, depressed, stuck, or overwhelmed. In this chapter, we look at how it can help caregivers manage their more difficult feelings.

Before you dive in, I want to set expectations: the goal here is not to force yourself into positivity. It's to build confidence that you can feel what you feel and still keep going. And when you're ready, you can also learn how to shift what is happening inside you so the hard moments don't knock you down as much.

Feel first.

Then change if you want.

Let's see how that works.

How CBT Works

At its core, CBT teaches one simple, life-changing idea: most of the time, it's not the situation itself that creates how you feel; it's what your mind says about the situation.

Let me show you what I mean.

Imagine you are at the grocery store and you see someone you know.

You wave.

They don't wave back. How would you feel?

When I ask this question in a room full of people, I never get one answer. I get a range.

Some people say angry.

Some say sad.

Some say worried.

Some say relieved.

Some feel nothing at all.

Same situation. Different feelings.

So what explains the difference? It's the thought.

The person who feels angry might be thinking, "They are ignoring me."

The person who feels sad might be thinking, "No one ever notices me."

The person who feels worried might be thinking, "They look distracted. I hope they're okay."

The person who feels relieved might be thinking, "Good. I didn't want to stop and talk today."

The person who feels neutral might be thinking, "They probably didn't see me."

Nothing about the situation changed.

The thought did. And the feeling followed.

Thoughts Create Feelings

This thought–feeling connection has been happening your entire life, even if you've never noticed it before. Most people move through life believing their situations create their feelings. And it certainly feels that way.

Your loved one lashes out and you feel hurt.

The doctor rushes through your questions and you feel dismissed.

The bills stack up and you feel overwhelmed.

Here is how it usually goes:

Something happens.

You feel something immediately.

You assume what happened caused the feeling.

But if that were true, we would all feel the same way about the same situations, but we don't.

Automatic Thoughts

We don't all react the same way to the same movie. Or the same music. Or the same decision someone else makes.

What is actually happening is this:

1. A situation happens.
2. Your brain offers an automatic thought about it.
3. That thought creates the feeling.

It's called an *automatic thought* because it shows up fast. So fast that you may not even realize it's there unless you look for it.

Why does this matter? Because it means that when you want to feel differently, you often have to think differently. It sounds simple, but it's not always easy.

It's one thing to practice this with a grocery store example.

It's another thing to practice it in the middle of dementia caregiving.

So let's bring it closer to home. Imagine you decide to move your loved one into a memory care facility. How do you imagine you would feel?

When I ask caregivers this question, I hear a wide range of answers too. Sad. Guilty. Anxious. Relieved.

Again, the situation is the same. The thoughts are different.

Sad might come from "I don't want to be away from them."

Guilt might come from "I should've been able to keep them at home."

Anxiety might come from "They aren't going to treat him well."

Relief might come from "I'm finally going to be able to rest."

This is one of the most important shifts you can make as a caregiver.

In most situations, you can't control what's happening around you. But you can influence what's happening inside you.

There are exceptions. If your life is in immediate danger, your brain and body respond on instinct. That is not the moment for thought work. But in most everyday moments, this thought–feeling connection is happening whether you notice it or not.

And this is actually good news.

Because if you don't like how you feel, you can often change it by changing the thought.

We can't change what already happened.

But we can change how we respond to what has already happened.

Where Your Control Still Lives

If you've ever been asked the same question over and over, you know how quickly it can wear on you. One Careblazer shared that her husband would ask the same question repeatedly throughout the day. At first, her thought was, *He is driving me crazy*. And with that came tension, frustration, and the urge to shut it down.

Over time, she began practicing a different thought: his brain is having a hard time holding on to the answer.

Nothing about the situation changed. The question still came. Again and again. But her response began to shift. She would answer the question and move on, instead of getting pulled into the frustration. It started to feel more like answering any other question, rather than something she needed to stop.

Another Careblazer found her own way of softening these moments. When her husband asked the same question, she started making a quiet game out of it. She would guess how many times he would ask, then smile to herself when she got close.

The question didn't stop. But the experience of it changed. It felt a little lighter to carry.

When you start to see your thoughts as the bridge between what is happening and how you feel, you unlock something powerful. In a situation where so much feels out of your control, it matters to know where you still have control.

You cannot control dementia.

You cannot control other people.

You cannot control what's already happened.

But you do have influence over how you respond.

I know this might sound simple.

I also know it's not easy.

Especially when you are exhausted, stressed, sleep-deprived, and already doing too much.

This is not meant to become another job on your to-do list.

You do not need to turn every hard feeling into an assignment.

Key Takeaways

- We can't control what has already happened, but we can choose how we think about it.
- Understanding the connection between our thoughts and feelings helps us see that situations themselves aren't forcing us to feel one specific way.
- Uncomfortable feelings don't always need to be changed. Sometimes they are exactly what makes sense to feel given what is happening.

Looking Ahead

Sometimes you just need to feel what you feel and let it move through you. But if there is a part of you wishing things felt a little easier, if there is a part of you that wants more emotional breathing room, this is a tool you can use.

Not to change every thought. But to notice when certain thoughts are making things heavier than they need to be, and to choose differently when you are ready.

Because when you understand the thought–feeling connection, you also begin to see something else. How you feel affects what you do. And what you do often affects how your loved one responds.

So before I teach you how to shift thoughts in a way that actually works, we need to talk about a few common traps that keep caregivers stuck when they first learn about the thought–feeling connection.

We'll talk about that in Chapter 5.

Chapter 5

Thoughts That Keep Us Stuck

Before we go any further, it's important to talk about some of the ways the thought–feeling connection can get misunderstood. Once you learn about this connection, it's easy for new pressure to sneak in. This pressure is often well-intentioned, but it can quietly add guilt, frustration, and self-criticism instead of relief.

It usually sounds something like this: if my thoughts affect how I feel, then I should be able to control my thoughts better.

This chapter will walk through some of the common ways our thinking can get in the way of using this approach.

One important note first: Sometimes situations can be violent or feel on the verge of violence at any moment. If you are in such a moment, changing your thoughts about the situation (such as CBT practice) is not what to focus on right then. In those situations, safety and outside support come first. Thought work can be helpful later, but not when your safety is at risk.

Myth 1: "I Should Think Positive All the Time"

Once you understand that thoughts influence feelings, it can be tempting to believe you should always be thinking positive thoughts.

And when you're not, your mind might go straight to thoughts such as these:

Why am I still feeling this way?

I should be better at this by now.

I must be doing it wrong.

Let's stop that right here.

Yes, your thoughts influence your feelings. But you are not making up this situation. Dementia is real. Caregiving is real life. And real life includes grief, resentment, exhaustion, anger, and heartbreak.

We often hear stories about caregivers who speak only about love, gratitude, and devotion. And while those stories can be true, they are incomplete.

I have worked with thousands of caregivers, and I have yet to meet one who has never had a negative thought about the person they care for. Not one.

No one thinks positive thoughts all the time. Negative thoughts do not mean you are a bad caregiver. They do not mean you are selfish. They do not mean you love your loved one any less. They mean you are human.

You may have thoughts that surprise you. You may not like your loved one all the time. You may feel frustrated, resentful, angry, or trapped. That doesn't make you cruel. It makes sense given how hard this is.

So if your thoughts do not sound like a Hallmark movie, nothing has gone wrong.

Myth 2: "If I Change My Thoughts, I'm Letting Them Get Away with It"

When caregivers learn that thoughts shape feelings, it can feel unfair.

Like this is one more thing you have to work on. One more adjustment you have to make. Even though you're already doing so much, and your loved one is the one being hurtful, unkind, or impossible to reason with.

This gets even more complicated when your relationship history is painful.

Some caregivers tell me:

- "He was always stubborn."
- "She was never kind to me."
- "If only you knew him, you would understand."

And they're right. History matters.

Here's what can get confused: caregivers sometimes think, "if I choose a thought that hurts less, then I'm excusing what happened. I'm pretending it was okay." That is not what this is.

Letting go of a painful thought is not approval. It is not permission. It is not rewriting history. It is choosing not to keep hurting yourself with the same story on repeat.

I once worked with a Careblazer who carried deep resentment toward her husband. Years before dementia, he had betrayed her. When dementia entered the picture, that old pain came roaring back.

Every act of caregiving felt loaded. Every sacrifice felt unfair. Her resentment made sense.

But it was also making caregiving unbearable.

The question was never whether her feelings were justified. They were.

The question was whether carrying them this way was helping her survive the day she was already living.

She began noticing an automatic thought that showed up every time she helped him: "He never loved me."

Those thoughts added to her resentment. And that resentment lived in her body all day long.

Over time, she practiced a different thought. One that didn't deny the past, but also didn't reopen the wound every time she showed up to care.

Something like: "I don't have to relive the past at this moment."

The past didn't disappear. But she stopped bleeding from it every single day.

Changing a thought does not erase accountability. It reduces your suffering.

On the surface, it might look like you're doing this to protect the person with dementia. But most of the time, you're doing it to protect you. You're the one carrying the anger, resentment, and grief in your body.

Myth 3: "I Shouldn't Change My Thought Because It's True"

Some of the most painful thoughts caregivers have are completely true.

I wish this were easier.

This should not be happening.

They would never do this for me.

"True" does not always mean helpful. A thought can be true and still make your life much harder. Repeating a painful truth over and over doesn't make it more true. It just makes it heavier.

This work is not about lying to yourself. It's about choosing thoughts that help you keep going without burning out.

It's true that I didn't always show up at my best while caring for my mom and dad. But replaying that on repeat doesn't change the past. It just steals strength from the present.

Myth 4: "This Won't Work for Me"

This thought and many like it are one of the fastest ways to get stuck.

This won't work for me.

I've tried everything.

Nothing makes a difference.

When your mind lands here, it stops looking for options.

Energy drops. Curiosity disappears. And ironically, this thought almost guarantees you won't get results, because you've already decided it won't.

The goal isn't to force yourself to believe something unrealistic. It's to practice a thought that leaves the door cracked open. For example:

I don't know yet what will help, but I'm willing to keep looking.

This might not fix everything, but it could help something.

One day I might find something that helps.

Hope doesn't have to be big to be powerful. It just has to keep you trying.

Myth 5: "I Can't Just Stop My Thoughts"

Thoughts are habits. Think about that. Many of the thoughts you have now have been playing on repeat for years:

I'm not good enough.

Everyone seems to have it easier than me.

Life isn't fair.

This is too hard.

Many of us carry a handful of thoughts that repeat in our minds for years, sometimes so often that we stop noticing them.

They are not going to disappear just because you noticed them.

And they don't necessarily need to. The goal isn't to stop or change every thought.

The goal is to notice them and decide whether you want to keep building that thought habit.

You don't have to win an argument with your thoughts. Just being aware of them can create space.

For example, imagine your loved one asks the same question again, a question you've already answered several times today. A thought might flash through your mind: *I shouldn't have to keep answering this.*

That thought naturally brings frustration with it. Most of us only notice the frustration. We don't pause long enough to notice the thought that came just before it.

But when you begin to recognize the thought itself, something shifts. You are no longer completely inside the frustration. You are noticing it.

From there, nothing else has to change. You may still feel irritated. The question may still come again. But simply being aware of the thought can loosen its grip a little.

And sometimes that awareness opens the door to another way of thinking about the moment. You might notice a different thought arise: *This is a cruel disease.* Or *His brain is struggling to hold on to information.*

We can create new habit thoughts that help us, rather than keep us frustrated.

Key Takeaways

- You don't have to think positive thoughts all the time. Difficult thoughts and feelings are part of being human, especially in a situation as hard as dementia caregiving.
- Changing a thought doesn't mean you are excusing what happened or pretending something was okay. It means you are choosing not to keep hurting yourself with the same story on repeat.
- A thought can be true and still make your life harder. Repeating painful truths over and over doesn't change the past. It only adds weight to the present.
- The goal is not to control every thought. The goal is to notice them and decide whether you want to choose to continue building the habit of that thought.

Looking Ahead

Sometimes just noticing a thought is enough to take away some of its power.

And if you do want to change a thought, you can learn how to do that too—without forcing positivity or pretending things are fine.

In Chapter 6, I'll walk you step-by-step through how to shift thoughts in a way that actually works.

Chapter 6

How to Actually Feel Better

Let's talk about how to actually feel better. But before we do, it's important to understand, feeling better doesn't mean feeling good about dementia. We can feel better without everything *being* better. That's important to say now.

As we talked about in previous chapters, if you want to feel better, you usually have to think thoughts that feel better.

Let's get started.

Believing Your Thoughts

We can't just say new sentences to ourselves and expect our feelings to magically change. That's the tricky part. The mind just doesn't work that way. This is not a fake-it-'til-you-make-it thing. This is a believe-it-so-you-can-feel-it thing.

Trying to think something you don't believe will not help. In fact, it often makes things worse. A thought can sound nice to your ears and still feel awful in the rest of your body.

Let me show you what I mean.

Imagine that it's been a long day. You lost your patience with your loved one. Dinner ended up being a bowl of cereal. You catch yourself daydreaming about a time when caregiving doesn't require so much mental gymnastics just to get through the day.

Then a familiar thought shows up: *I'm a bad caregiver*.

You notice that thought makes you feel guilty.

After learning that thoughts shape feelings, you decide you don't want to feel guilty anymore. So you try to replace that thought with *I'm an amazing caregiver.*

But chances are, that jump doesn't work.

If you don't actually believe you are an amazing caregiver, that thought will feel hollow. Your mind will immediately argue with it. And instead of relief, you may feel even worse.

This is a really important point. It doesn't matter how good a thought sounds.

What matters is how good it feels.

For a thought to shift how you feel, you have to be able to believe it.

The Belief Bridge

This is where something I call the *belief bridge* can help.

Instead of trying to leap from *I'm a bad caregiver* straight to *I'm an amazing caregiver*, you build a bridge between those two thoughts.

That bridge might sound like these thoughts:

It's possible I'm not a bad caregiver.

I'm working on becoming a good caregiver.

There are moments when I am a good caregiver.

These bridge thoughts might not ultimately be what you want to believe right now, but over time, those thoughts may naturally lead you to believe *I am an amazing caregiver.*

Your belief doesn't have to change all at once.

And it doesn't have to change today. Your only job is to take the next step that feels believable.

Every step across that bridge matters, because each step creates a small shift in how you feel. And those small shifts add up.

And before you judge yourself for any of this, let me say something clearly: if you lost your patience recently or dinner ended up being cereal, that doesn't mean you are a bad caregiver. Most of the time, it means you are exhausted and carrying a lot.

Why This Works in the Brain

Here's the simple version of what is happening in your brain: your mind is very good at finding evidence for whatever you already believe. If you believe you are a bad caregiver, your brain will quickly notice every snapped comment, every forgotten task, every imperfect moment. It will replay them on a loop.

At the same time, it will quietly minimize or dismiss evidence that does not fit that belief. Things like the fact that you are reading this book. That you show up day after day. That you keep trying.

In psychology, this is known as *confirmation bias*. Your brain confirms what you believe, whether it's actually true or not.

When you begin practicing more balanced, believable thoughts, your brain slowly starts noticing different evidence. Not because reality changed, but because your focus did.

This is not about tricking yourself. It is about widening what your mind allows you to see.

The Thought Swap

So what do you actually do when you want to feel better? First, as a reminder, you *always* feel first. You never skip that step.

Okay, here is a simple process I call the *thought swap*.

Once you recognize an uncomfortable feeling, ask yourself this question:

1. Do I want to feel this way?

If yes, stop here.

If not:

2. How would I like to feel instead?

3. What thought might help me feel even a little closer to that?

That is it.

No forcing.

No pressure.

No requirement that you do this every time.

Think of new thoughts the way you think of trying on shoes. Some look great on the shelf, but the moment you put them on, they pinch or rub the wrong way.

A thought only works if it feels better in your body. If it does, keep it.

If it doesn't, try another.

Do this even if the thought doesn't sound particularly pretty. I once worked with a woman who was caring for her mother. Their relationship had always been strained. Her mother had not shown up for her when she needed support most.

The caregiver told me, "I'm doing this because if I don't, no one will."

That thought was true. But it made her feel deeply resentful.

We explored whether there was another honest reason she was showing up. After some time, she said, "I think I'm doing this because I'm a better person than she was to me."

That thought may not sound pretty. But when I asked how it felt, she said, "It makes me feel proud."

Both thoughts were true, but one created resentment and the other created pride.

That is the power of choosing thoughts based on how they feel, not how they sound.

When You Don't Want to Change Your Thoughts

Just because you can change something doesn't mean you always have to. Sometimes, even with all of this, you are tired.

> You don't want to work on your thoughts.
>
> You don't want another tool.
>
> You just want to get through the day.

That is okay. You have options.

You can feel your feelings and do nothing else at all. You can notice a thought without changing it.

Or you can decide to work with it.

None of these choices are wrong.

The Thought Buffet

If you do decide you want to try on another thought, here is a metaphor that many of my Careblazers find helpful.

Your mind is always offering you a buffet of thoughts. Some are nourishing. Some will make you feel sick.

> You don't have control over everything that shows up on the buffet.
>
> But you do get to choose what you keep piling onto your plate.

Continuing to focus on thoughts you know make you feel awful is like filling your plate with liver when your favorite food of mashed potatoes is right there.

You can set the plate down.

You can grab a new one.

You can choose again.

This is not easy work. Especially when you have been thinking the same thoughts for years.

But the only thing harder than learning how to work with your thoughts is continuing to carry the ones that are keeping you stuck.

Key Takeaways

- Thoughts only change feelings when you actually believe them. A thought that sounds nice but feels untrue will not help.
- Real change usually happens in small steps. Bridge thoughts help you move gradually from a painful belief to one that feels more supportive.
- Your brain naturally looks for evidence that confirms what you already believe. When your thoughts shift, what your mind notices begins to shift, too.
- You don't have to force yourself to think a "perfect" thought. The goal is that the thought feels a little better and believable to you.
- Sometimes the most helpful thoughts are not the prettiest ones. What matters is how the thought makes you feel, not how it sounds.

Looking Ahead

Of course, some thoughts are more negative than others. These thoughts can be difficult to either sit with or change.

In Chapter 7, we talk about the common feelings that weigh caregivers down the most. Guilt. Self-judgment. And the quiet stories that tell you that you are never doing enough.

Chapter 7

So What Does This Mean for Behaviors?

You might be wondering why we've spent so much time talking about thoughts and feelings in a book about managing dementia-related behaviors.

That's a fair question. Here's the simple answer: the more frustrated you feel, the more frustrating caregiving becomes. The more anxious you feel, the more anxiety shows up in the day. The more overwhelmed you feel, the harder everything feels to manage.

This is not because you're doing something wrong. It's because how you feel shapes how you show up.

This chapter is not about asking you to do more all the time. It's about helping you gain a sense of control in a situation that takes so much of it away.

The Situation and the Experience

When a challenging behavior happens, who do you think is more likely to get through the moment with less damage to the relationship and to themselves: a caregiver who feels tense, resentful, and overwhelmed or a caregiver who feels calmer, more grounded, and more confident?

Most of us move between both, sometimes in the same day.

The situation might be the same, but it feels different. When you feel less on edge, it's easier to stay steady, think more clearly, and respond in a way that doesn't make things harder.

This doesn't mean you need to feel good all the time. And it certainly doesn't mean your feelings are to blame for your loved one's behavior. It means understanding that your thoughts drive your feelings, and your feelings shape how you respond.

So far, we have learned this sequence:

1. A situation happens.
2. Your mind offers a thought.
3. That thought creates a feeling.
4. That feeling influences your actions.
5. And your actions affect how your loved one responds.

How you feel matters because it shapes what you say, how you say it, what you try, and what you stop trying.

A frustrated caregiver speaks differently than a calm caregiver.

A resentful caregiver reacts differently than a compassionate caregiver.

An exhausted caregiver problem-solves differently than a supported one.

You have probably noticed this already. You have likely seen moments where your tone, your body language, or your emotional state made a situation escalate or soften.

That is not a failure.

That is being human in a very hard situation.

This is why the most effective way to manage difficult moments often starts with managing our own response first.

Managing Your Response

It can feel deeply unfair to hear that you have to change your response. You are already doing so much.

You did not cause the disease.

You did not ask for this role.

And yet here we are, talking about one more thing that involves you adjusting.

It is okay to feel frustrated about that. The truth is, we don't work on ourselves because it's fair.

We do it because it helps.

You can't control dementia. You can't control how your loved one's brain is changing. You can't control what behaviors will show up tomorrow.

But you do have influence over how you respond. And that influence matters.

I imagine it might be frustrating that so much of what makes caregiving easier requires more change and effort from you. That's the part no one wants to hear.

I also want to be very clear about something: even when you respond thoughtfully and with care, your loved one may still feel agitated, distressed, or confused. Just as we can't protect all the people we love from every uncomfortable feeling, we cannot protect someone with dementia from them either.

But—and this is the part that matters most to me—while your thoughts and feelings can influence your loved one's behavior, my true hope is that this work helps *you* feel better.

Yes, in many cases it will help interactions go more smoothly. But even when it does not, it can still reduce your suffering.

The worst-case scenario is that your loved one continues to show difficult dementia-related behaviors, but you feel better while it's happening. Because at the heart of dementia caregiving, the most important factor is you.

The most effective way to improve dementia care is to support the caregiver. You are the one providing care.

Advocating.

Problem-solving.

Showing up day after day.

And life doesn't pause because someone you love has dementia. You still have responsibilities, relationships, bills, appointments, and obligations. Everything keeps moving, even when you feel frozen.

Up to this point, the goal has been to help you understand why this feels so hard and to remind you there are ways to ease the pain.

Key Takeaways

- How you feel in a moment influences how you show up. And how you show up often shapes what happens next.
- The most powerful place to begin changing difficult moments is often not the behavior, but your own response to it.
- You cannot control dementia or every behavior that appears, but you do have influence over how you respond when it happens.

Looking Ahead

The chapters in Part II focus on practical tools to help make daily life easier to face.

Now that you understand why your inner world matters so much, we can move into the practical strategies that help you respond more effectively in the moments that matter most.

That is where we go next.

The strategies in the coming chapters are not magic tricks. They do not fix dementia. They reduce friction, suffering, and unnecessary escalation. And they work best when you're not already pushed past your limit.

This is where the inner work meets the practical work.

Part II

The Strategies: Focusing on the Person with Dementia

Chapter 8

Your Dementia Behavior Toolkit

In Part I, we looked at how dementia-related behaviors can feel unpredictable, frustrating, and exhausting.

And while dementia itself cannot be fixed, there *are* ways to make daily caregiving feel more manageable.

We've spent time talking about understanding why dementia-related behaviors happen and why it feels so hard emotionally. Now it's time to talk about what to do with that information. Sympathy is nice. Strategies are even better.

Part II focuses on practical strategies you can use to respond to behaviors with more confidence and less stress.

A Caregiving Toolkit

Think of what follows as tools, not rules. Use what helps in the situation you're facing, and set aside what doesn't. These strategies fall into five key categories:

- **Success strategies for any behavior:** Here are some core approaches that apply to almost every behavior and make all other strategies more effective.
- **Proactive strategies for success:** There are some things you can do ahead of time to reduce the chance that certain behaviors happen at all.

- **In-the-moment strategies:** Here are some tools to help you respond when something is already unfolding and emotions are running high.
- **Communication strategies:** Small shifts in how you speak and respond can dramatically change how well your loved one understands you.
- **Strategies for adapting to their reality:** As dementia changes the brain, our approaches have to change, too. This section helps you adjust along the way.

Every strategy in this section has been used successfully by caregivers in real life. These aren't ideas that just sound good on paper. They are approaches that have helped caregivers calm situations more quickly, reduce stress, and in many cases prevent certain behaviors altogether.

Think of this section as a caregiving toolkit.

Just as you would not use the same tool for every household repair, you will not use the same strategy for every behavior. That is why you will find a variety of options here.

Some of these strategies may help in big ways. Others may help in smaller ways. And some may not fit your situation at all. That doesn't mean you're doing anything wrong. And if something doesn't work today, it doesn't mean you failed. It simply means you may need a different tool tomorrow.

As you read, try not to focus too much on the exact situation being described. Instead, pay attention to how the caregiver responds. Each strategy can be adapted to many different situations, not just the example given.

At the end of each strategy, you will find prompts to help you apply it to your own situation.

Some of these approaches may feel brand-new. Others may sound familiar. If you catch yourself thinking, *I've tried this before*, pause and ask a different question: *How might this look now, with everything I've learned so far?*

The mindset work you have already done matters here. It will shape how effective these strategies feel and how confident you are using them.

Key Takeaways

- While we may not be able to stop or prevent every dementia-related behavior, using the right strategies at the right time can reduce stress and help situations feel less overwhelming.
- You may not use every strategy, and you won't use the same strategy every time. If something doesn't work, it simply means a different tool may be needed.
- Caregiving requires flexibility. What works today may not work tomorrow, and that's a normal part of adjusting to a changing reality.

Looking Ahead

As you begin to work through the chapters ahead, please keep the following in mind:

First, you do not need to read this section in order. You are welcome to jump around, revisit chapters, and come back to strategies as things change.

Also, and this is important: remember, this is not about doing everything perfectly.

It is about giving yourself more options.

Let's begin.

Chapter 9

Success Strategies for Any Behavior

Dementia-related behaviors can look like a lot of different things. Care that suddenly feels hard. Eating becoming complicated. Questions repeating over and over. Emotions surfacing in ways that feel sudden, confusing, or out of character. While the situations may look different, the way you respond often matters more than the specific behavior itself.

This chapter introduces a set of core strategies that can be used across many different dementia-related behaviors. They are not tied to one specific situation. They are ways of thinking and responding that you can return to again and again, no matter what shows up day-to-day.

The strategies in this chapter are meant to give you more options in those moments. As you read, there is a good chance you will recognize something you are dealing with right now. And there is likely at least one approach here you can start trying immediately.

This is not about getting it right every time or stopping every behavior. It is about reducing stress, easing tension, and avoiding unnecessary power struggles. When that shifts, caregiving feels more manageable, and your loved one often feels calmer, too.

Remember: you do not need to remember all of these strategies. This is not a checklist. It is a collection of options you can return to as things change.

It may be most helpful to read through this chapter with curiosity rather than pressure. Notice which approaches stand out to you or feel like they might fit your situation. You can mark those and come back to them later, when you are ready to think more about how they might apply to what you are dealing with right now.

Focus on the Ending, Not Their Understanding

When someone has dementia, their ability to understand what is happening is often unreliable. They may not be able to understand they need help. They may not understand what's happening around them. They may believe things that aren't true.

That doesn't mean they're being stubborn or difficult. It means their brain may no longer be able to process, store, or trust the information we are trying to give them.

Have you ever found yourself stuck in an argument with your loved one, desperately trying to prove something that feels so obvious, but no matter what you say, they just won't believe you?

It's frustrating, right?

Now imagine what would happen if you stopped trying to convince them and instead focused on what you needed to happen next.

That's exactly what one of my Care Collective members, Sally, learned when she was running errands with her mom, who has dementia. The day had gone smoothly until they pulled into the driveway. Sally told her mom, "We're home!" But her mom didn't believe it.

"This isn't my house," her mom insisted, refusing to get out of the car.

Sally did what most of us would do. She tried to prove reality. She pulled out the car registration, showed her mom the address, even pulled up photos of the house on her phone. But instead of reassuring her mom, this just made her mom more upset.

That's because convincing doesn't work when the brain can no longer reliably process new information or update beliefs.

The harder we try to force understanding, the more distress we often create.

Instead of trying to get her mom to understand, Sally needed to focus on the ending: getting her mom out of the car and inside the house.

The goal wasn't agreement. The goal was getting her out of the car and into the home.

Here are some different approaches:

- "This is our last stop; thanks so much for helping me today!"
- "Let's go inside and grab a drink. I'm thirsty."
- "Last errand of the day; we did it!"

These responses don't argue. They don't force reality. They simply guide the situation toward the goal. None of them required her mom to accept that it was her house.

We don't need the person with dementia to understand what we understand. We don't need them to agree to our reality. What we *do* need is to focus on the goal.

> **Bonus Tip:** If your loved one enjoys something specific—gardening, music, a favorite TV show—use that to your advantage. In Sally's case, her mom loved gardening. A simple response like "I hear this house has a beautiful garden. Let's go take a look!" could have worked surprisingly well.

This approach is especially powerful when someone with dementia is experiencing delusions (believing things that aren't true) or visual hallucinations (seeing things that aren't there).

Instead of trying to correct them or prove them wrong (both of which will only increase frustration), focus on the ending you want and ask yourself, *What can I do or say to make that outcome more likely?*

> **Care in Action:** The next time you feel the urge to convince your loved one of something, pause. Instead of focusing on their understanding of the situation, focus on the ending you want. What can you say or do to get closer to that outcome?

Focus on Understanding Before Changing

When a behavior feels disruptive, frustrating, or confusing, it's natural to want to stop it. But if we rush to fix the behavior without first trying to understand it, we miss valuable clues that could help us reduce the behavior or prevent it from happening again. We also miss what they actually need. And the behaviors usually continue. Sometimes they even get worse.

Take Terry, for example. She recently joined our Care Collective program and shared that her mother screamed every night in her bedroom. This was deeply stressful for Terry and her entire family. No one was getting sleep.

At first, Terry focused on stopping the screaming. Every night, when her mom screamed, she rushed into the room to comfort her. She reassured her mom that everything was okay, that there was nothing to be scared of, and asked her mom to calm down.

But none of it worked. Terry couldn't get her mom to understand everything was okay.

By focusing only on stopping the behavior, Terry wasn't looking for clues. She wasn't considering what might be triggering the screaming or what her mother was experiencing in that moment.

But once Terry shifted her focus to understanding before changing, she started noticing details she hadn't before. That's when she saw it. Her mom looked scared. And the bed was facing a large mirrored closet.

Terry wondered: *Could her mom be frightened by her own reflection, mistaking it for a stranger?*

She decided to turn the bed away from the mirror.

The screaming stopped.

Nothing about her mother changed. The environment did.

Had Terry continued focusing only on stopping the behavior, she'd still be rushing into the room every night, offering comfort that didn't solve the real problem. Even worse, her mom would still be experiencing fear, night after night.

It's important to remember that the behaviors that cause stress and frustration for caregivers are just as distressing for the person with dementia. These behaviors are a form of communication. Our job as dementia detectives is to uncover what they're trying to tell us.

Here are some questions to guide your detective work. You can ask them in the moment when possible, or later when things are calm.

- What might they be trying to communicate or solve?
- What emotion might be driving this right now (fear, confusion, embarrassment, frustration, pain)?
- What exactly are they doing, step-by-step (and what need could that represent)?
- When is this behavior not happening? What is different then?
- What happened right before it started (time of day, noise, lighting, people, demands, hunger, fatigue)?
- Where is their attention focused during the behavior?

Instead of reacting with frustration, approach behaviors with curiosity. Not only will this shift help you feel more in control as a caregiver, but it will also help your loved one feel safer and more understood.

> **Care in Action:** The next time a behavior shows up, pause before you try to stop it. Ask yourself, *What might this be communicating?* Then look for one small clue.

You may not have the answer in the heat of the moment, but by reviewing the situation afterward and looking for clues, you'll start to see patterns and solutions you might have otherwise missed.

See the "Remove or Replace Triggers" section in Chapter 10 for another solution that could've worked nicely in this situation.

Assess Don't Assume

Sometimes, what we assume is the problem isn't the problem at all. That's why the Assess Don't Assume strategy is so important.

Here's a scenario: Jenny's mom started pulling tissues out of the box, tossing them onto the floor, and then placing the empty box on her feet. To Jenny, this seemed wasteful—her mom was throwing perfectly good tissues on the ground!

Frustrated, she told her mom to stop. When that didn't work, she took the tissue box away.

Her mom became upset. Jenny was just doing what she thought was right, stopping her mom from wasting tissues.

But was her mom *really* "wasting" tissues? Or was she doing something else?

It's easy to assume we know what's happening when a person with dementia behaves in a way that seems illogical or frustrating.

From Jenny's perspective, her mom was simply being wasteful. And most people would probably agree—her mom *was* wasting tissue!

But when we look at the situation from Jenny's mom's perspective, we realize that's not true at all.

Instead of assuming, Jenny paused. She stepped back and assessed. That's when she noticed something she hadn't before—her mom wasn't just pulling tissues out randomly. She kept placing the empty tissue box on her feet.

Then it clicked. Jenny wondered: *Could her mom's feet be cold?*

She brought her mom a pair of socks, and, just like that, the behavior stopped.

Her mom wasn't trying to waste tissues. She was trying to meet an unspoken need in the only way she could.

Many "difficult" behaviors are messages. But when we assume we already know what's happening, we risk responding in ways that don't address the real issue.

If Jenny had continued to assume her mom was just wasting tissues, she would have focused only on stopping the behavior by taking the tissues away, while her mom's feet remained cold.

When we assess rather than assume, we become more curious, more observant, and more open to solutions that actually work.

Here are things that are *never* helpful when responding to difficult behavior:

- Assuming the person is acting out on purpose to upset you.
- Believing "They've always been difficult—this is just them being them."
- Arguing with them about what they're doing or why they shouldn't be doing it.

Care in Action: Is there a dementia-related behavior that has you stumped? Take a step back. Pause. Put aside your assumptions and get curious.

Ask yourself:

What might they be trying to communicate?

Could they be feeling discomfort, frustration, or fear?

What environmental factors could be playing a role?

What small change could I make to see if it helps?

Use your answers to guide your next step—and you may just uncover a simple, effective solution.

Kindness over Truth

For many of us, telling the truth feels like the right thing to do.

But in dementia care, the truth can sometimes cause more harm than help.

Take driving, for example. If a person with dementia is no longer safe to drive, reminding them of that fact every time they mention driving will not change their reality. What it often changes is how unsafe or upset the interaction feels for both of you.

Many people with dementia struggle to remember or accept their limitations. For some, memory loss makes it impossible to recall that they can no longer drive. For others, *anosognosia* (discussed in Chapter 2) prevents them from recognizing their impairments at all. This looks exactly like denial, but it isn't a choice.

In either case, repeatedly telling the truth does not lead to understanding. It leads to distress. Because their brain has trouble storing new information, each reminder can feel like hearing the news for the first time.

So what can you do instead? This is where the Kindness over Truth approach comes in. Rather than defaulting to the most factual response, ask yourself, *What is the kindest response right now?*

Let's look at the driving example again.

A truthful response might be:

- "You are not safe to drive anymore."
- "Your license was taken away."
- "You have dementia and can't drive."

All of these statements are factually correct.

None of them are likely to help.

A kinder response might sound like:

- "You always loved driving."
- "Tell me about your favorite car."
- "You drove me everywhere. I like getting to do that for you now."
- "I will be your chauffeur today" (while opening the passenger door).

Sometimes, the kindest response is not verbal at all. You might:

- Listen without correcting.
- Disable the car.
- Remove visual triggers like car keys or parking in the driveway.

The goal isn't to correct them.

And it isn't to lie.

It's to respond in a way that prevents unnecessary distress.

Here is another common situation: a person with dementia asks about someone who has passed away. Because they don't remember the death, each reminder can feel like losing that person all over again.

Here are some truthful responses:

- "They passed away."
- "Remember, they died last year."

While these statements are true, they often cause repeated emotional pain.

A kinder response might be:

- "They're not here right now."
- "You really miss them."
- "I think I have some photos. Let's look at them together."

These responses do not deny feelings. They acknowledge them and shift the focus in a compassionate way.

One of the hardest adjustments in dementia care is learning that connection often matters more than correction.

In everyday conversations, we answer questions directly. We clarify misunderstandings. We rely on facts. Dementia often requires a different approach, one that prioritizes emotional safety over accuracy.

Kindness over Truth does not mean withholding important information forever. People with dementia do need to be told difficult truths at certain points.

This approach is about recognizing when information is not being remembered or believed and understanding that repeating it only creates more pain.

Care in Action: The next time you feel the urge to correct or remind your loved one of a fact you know will upset them, pause.

Ask yourself:

- *Does this question actually need a factual answer?*
- *What emotion might be underneath it?*
- *Is there a kinder way to respond?*

Even if the response doesn't feel like a direct answer, try it and see what happens. Many caregivers are surprised by how much calmer and more connected their interactions become when kindness, not necessarily the truth, leads the way.

Respond to the Emotion, Not the Words

Sometimes a person with dementia will say things that don't make sense or are simply not true. They might insist someone is breaking into the house when no one is there, or believe they are still safe to drive when they are not.

I once worked with a client who believed people were breaking into his home at night and changing his kitchen cabinets.

This is an example of a delusion: a strong, fixed belief that remains even when there is clear evidence to the contrary. In situations like this, arguing does not work. Reasoning does not work. Even proof does not work.

If I had shown him a video recording proving no one entered his home, he would have explained it away. His brain would have found a way to make what he believed the truth.

When he told me about the intruders, and after I confirmed there were in fact no intruders coming into the home, I had two options:

Option 1: Respond to his words: "No one is breaking into your home and changing your cabinets."

This response would likely have led to an argument, increased his frustration, and damaged trust.

Option 2: Respond to his emotion: "That sounds really upsetting to think someone is breaking into your home."

This response acknowledged how he felt without challenging what he believed.

By choosing the second option, the conversation stayed focused on his emotional experience rather than his delusion. That shift mattered. It avoided a power struggle and kept our trust.

It also enabled us to move the conversation toward one of the goals we were working on together: increasing his activity during the day and improving his sleep. Because we weren't stuck arguing about cabinets, we could focus on helping him feel calmer and safer.

Once you acknowledge the emotion, you can gently guide the moment in a more productive direction.

For example, if someone seems angry or scared, you might say,

- "You sound really upset. What do you usually do when you feel this way?"
- "When I feel upset, going for a walk helps me calm down. What about you?"
- "Let's try that together."

Notice what these responses do not do:

- They do not argue.
- They do not correct.
- They do not agree with something untrue.

They focus on emotion and help the person move forward.

There will also be moments when someone with dementia is faced with genuinely hard news, such as:

- Being told they can no longer drive.
- Learning they are moving into assisted living.
- Knowing they are getting worse.

In these moments, trying to convince them they should not feel upset is not realistic. Instead, you can simply acknowledge what they are feeling:

- "You sound sad."
- "Tell me more."
- "I'm sorry you're going through this."
- "I'm here with you."
- "What helps when you feel this way?"

When you respond to emotion rather than argue with their version of reality, you create a sense of safety. That safety often reduces distress on its own. Think about how helpful it feels to talk with a trusted friend who listens, even when they can't fix the situation.

People with dementia may live in a different reality, but their emotions are very real.

Correcting creates resistance.

Acknowledging creates connection.

Focusing on emotion gives you a way forward when logic fails.

From a brain perspective, this makes sense. The amygdala, the brain's emotional center, often remains active even as memory and reasoning decline. This means emotional responses are often more effective than factual ones.

> **Care in Action:** The next time your loved one is upset about something that is not true, try responding to the emotion behind their words instead of the words themselves.

If this feels uncomfortable at first, that is normal. Try it anyway and observe what happens.

- When they believe something that is not true:
  - "That sounds really frustrating."
  - "I can see why you would feel that way."
  - "That sounds upsetting. I'm here."
- When they insist they can still do something unsafe:
  - "I know how much driving meant to you."
  - "That independence was really important."
  - "Tell me about your favorite road trip."
  - "Let's go for a drive together, and I'll take the wheel."
- When they ask about someone who has passed away:
  - "You really miss them."
  - "They were such a big part of your life."

    - "Let's look at some pictures."
    - "Tell me a favorite memory."
- When they are upset about a major change:
    - "This is a lot to take in."
    - "I can see how hard this is."
    - "I'm here with you."
    - "We will take this one step at a time."

You do not need to fix the emotion.
You just need to meet it.

Use the "Right" Response

Caregivers often ask me, "Did I respond the right way?" They'll share a situation and wonder if their reaction was appropriate.

My answer is always the same: the best way to know if your response was the "right" one is by looking at your loved one's reaction, not mine.

- Did they seem calmer afterward?
- Did the situation de-escalate, even a little?
- Did it prevent things from getting worse?

There are no universally "right" or "wrong" responses in dementia care. What works for one person may completely backfire for another. Dementia affects individuals, not robots following a script. Every person brings their own history, personality, and preferences into the moment.

Tip: As you move forward and begin using the strategies in the coming pages, remember that the most reliable way to know whether an approach is helpful is to observe how your loved one responds.

If they become more distressed, it may mean that strategy is not a good fit for them. It may also mean the approach needs a small adjustment in timing, tone, or delivery.

If they seem calmer, more engaged, or recover more quickly, you are likely moving in the right direction.

The bottom line: your loved one's response is your most important feedback.

Care in Action: Each time you try a new approach, pay attention to what happens next. If it does not work the way you hoped, resist the urge to label it a failure. Instead, consider what you might tweak and try again. Small adjustments often lead to significant change.

Do Less to De-Escalate

Sometimes, the most effective response is hardly reacting at all.

When a challenging behavior happens, it can feel almost impossible to do nothing. Our instincts tell us to respond, explain, defend, or fix the situation immediately. But in some moments, especially during verbal accusations or emotional outbursts, the most effective response is not reacting at all.

I once witnessed a powerful example of this during a live video call with members of our Care Collective. While one caregiver was on the call, her husband, who has dementia, began yelling at her from across the room. He used vulgar language and accused her of lying. His voice was angry and loud. Everyone on the call could hear it.

Most of us braced ourselves, expecting her to react or disengage.

Instead, she looked at him calmly and said,

"I know, honey. I'm sorry. I'll get better, my love."

Then she turned back to the screen and continued to participate in our conversation as if nothing had happened.

It was a masterclass in responding without escalating.

Afterward, someone asked her, "How do you stay so calm?"

She answered without hesitation.

"That's not him."

She explained that the man yelling and calling her names was not the man she married. It was a man whose brain had been damaged by disease. Because she holds onto that belief, she does not feel the need to defend herself, correct him, or internalize what he says.

She had learned there was no benefit to arguing back.

No benefit to correcting.

And no benefit to letting his words seep into her sense of self.

During the rest of the call, her husband had several more accusatory outbursts. Each time, she responded the same way. Calm. Loving. Non-defensive. And each time, the moment passed without escalating.

It's easy to believe that when a behavior repeats, we must change our response. It's easy to believe that accusations require defense. It's easy to believe that silence means failure.

But sometimes, acknowledging without engaging is the most regulating response available.

Remember:

- Not every behavior needs an explanation.
- Not every accusation needs a defense.
- Not every moment requires action.

In some situations, doing less prevents the situation from becoming more.

This strategy is not about ignoring safety concerns or tolerating harm. If someone is at risk of being hurt, intervention is necessary. But when the behavior is verbal, repetitive, or emotionally driven, doing less can keep the moment from escalating.

Care in Action: The next time your loved one accuses you of something that isn't true or speaks in a way that feels hurtful, pause before reacting.

Instead of defending yourself, correcting, or redirecting, try continuing what you are doing while offering a brief, caring acknowledgment:

- "I'll get better."
- "I'm sorry, my love."
- "I know this feels frustrating."

Then let the moment pass.

Doing nothing does not mean you do not care.

Sometimes, it means you care enough not to add fuel to the fire.

Improv the Moment

This strategy is all about how to keep the conversation going instead of shutting it down.

Many caregivers tell me one of the most exhausting parts of dementia care is not knowing how to respond when their loved one says things that don't make sense.

They worry about saying the wrong thing. They feel pressure to correct inaccuracies. They feel frustrated when conversations seem to go nowhere.

One caregiver shared that she used to leave these conversations feeling irritated and drained. Her husband often said things that felt illogical or completely untrue, and she never knew how to respond without either correcting him or shutting down the conversation.

Then she did something unexpected: she signed up for an improv class.

Instead of trying to end conversations or force logic where it no longer existed, she learned how to go with them. And to her surprise, conversations that once felt frustrating started to feel lighter, more playful, and sometimes even enjoyable.

If you have ever watched improvisational comedy, you may have noticed some of the core rules of improv:

- You keep the scene going.
- You do not correct.
- You do not shut it down.
- You leave room for the other person to continue.

In many ways, people with dementia are already doing this. When their brain struggles to remember or make sense of information, it fills in the gaps. Sometimes that looks like believing a relative who passed away called earlier in the day. Sometimes it sounds nonsensical or untrue.

Our logical brain wants to step in and correct them.

- "That's not possible."
- "They passed away years ago."
- "That didn't happen."

But when we do that, we shut down the scene.

The conversation ends.

And frustration usually takes its place.

Improvising means keeping the door open.

If your loved one says a relative who passed away visited earlier, you might respond with:

- "Tell me more about that."
- "What did they have to say?"
- "That must have been nice."

These responses do not argue.

They do not correct.

They do not require the person with dementia to track facts they can no longer hold.

They allow your loved one to stay in their world. And when you do that, yours often becomes more peaceful, too.

This approach is especially helpful during casual conversation, storytelling, or moments where facts no longer matter but connection still does. Rather than focusing on what is factually true, you connect with what feels true to them in that moment. That connection matters more than accuracy.

The caregiver who shared this strategy told me that conversations she once dreaded became moments she could tolerate and sometimes even enjoy. Not because dementia had changed, but because her approach had.

She stopped trying to correct the conversation and started participating in it.

> **Care in Action:** The next time your loved one says something that doesn't make sense or is not true, pause before correcting.

Instead, try responding in a way that keeps the conversation going:

- Ask a curious question.
- Reflect interest.
- Invite them to share more.

Step Away

I once worked with a man who was becoming increasingly frustrated by his wife's repeated belief that the neighbors were changing things on their property. Each time she brought it up, he tried to convince her otherwise. He showed her videos. He explained. He reasoned.

And each time, both of them became more upset.

The more he tried to make her understand, the more stuck they both became.

That's when we talked about a different option, one that many caregivers forget they have: you are allowed to walk away.

You don't have to address everything the moment it comes up. You don't have to stay in a conversation that is going nowhere.

And you don't have to sacrifice your own emotional regulation to prove a point.

The next time his wife brought up the neighbors, instead of engaging, he practiced excusing *himself*.

- "I'll be right back, I forgot something."
- "I need to use the restroom."
- "Let me grab a glass of water."

Simple. Neutral. No confrontation.

By stepping away, he interrupted the escalation. When he returned later, the intensity of the belief had often passed. And even when it hadn't, *he* was calmer and better able to respond.

This is not giving up.

It's choosing not to pour energy into a situation that is only making things worse for everyone involved.

When you notice yourself getting pulled into a losing argument or feel your own frustration rising, stepping away can be the most regulating response for both of you.

> **Care in Action:** The next time a conversation starts to escalate, give yourself permission to pause it. Use a neutral excuse to step away and revisit the moment later, or not at all. You don't have to solve everything in real time. Sometimes the most effective response is not engaging at all.

Focus on Moving One Step Closer

Sometimes caregiving feels discouraging because you already know you won't get the end result you want.

You may want them to change their clothes, take a shower, eat a full meal, or cooperate with care, and because you can't see a clear path to that outcome, you stop trying altogether.

But caregiving is rarely about one big success. It's about small movements in the right direction.

A marathon is not completed in one stride. It is completed one step at a time. On any given day, one step may not feel like much. But over time, those steps build momentum, endurance, and meaningful change.

It's okay if the full goal doesn't happen today. The question to ask instead is, *Is there something I can do that moves us one step closer?*

If your loved one refuses to get into the shower, would a foot soak that feels like a pedicure help clean part of their body while keeping things calm?

If bathing feels impossible, could washing hands in a warm bowl of soapy water be framed as helping with dishes or cleaning silverware?

If hygiene is the concern but the bathroom is a barrier, could a bidet clean them while they sit on the toilet as you continue working toward a shower another day?

There are often many smaller options on the path to a larger goal. Do not dismiss them simply because they are not the ideal solution.

Remember:

- Partial care is *still* care.
- Reduced distress is *still* success.
- Progress *matters*.

When you allow yourself to aim for "one step closer" instead of "all or nothing," caregiving becomes more flexible, more humane, and far more sustainable.

Care in Action: The next time you feel stuck because the "best" outcome feels impossible, pause and ask yourself: *What would one small step toward that goal look like today?*

Then try that step, without judging it for not being perfect. Sometimes one step is exactly enough for today.

Bringing It All Together

These core approaches won't solve everything overnight. But they can shift the tone of your interactions, reduce your stress, and help your loved one feel more understood.

By now, you've learned how to do the following:

- Shift your focus from fixing behaviors to understanding them.
- Respond to emotions instead of arguing about facts.
- Choose kindness over correction.
- Look at what's really driving a behavior before reacting.

These are powerful tools.

They aren't just ways to get through the day.

They are ways to create more workable days.

And we're not stopping here. What if you could reduce the chances of certain behaviors happening in the first place?

In Chapter 10, we'll build on this foundation and look at proactive strategies you can use ahead of time. These approaches are designed to lower stress, reduce triggers, and make difficult moments less likely to escalate.

That's where we go next.

Chapter 10

Proactive Strategies for Success

Many dementia care strategies focus on what to do *after* a behavior has already started. That makes sense. Most caregivers are responding in real time, doing their best in the moment.

But there is another layer of support that often gets overlooked. Small changes made *before* a behavior starts can sometimes make the moment itself easier or keep it from escalating in the first place.

The strategies in this chapter focus on what you can adjust ahead of time to reduce friction, lower stress, and create conditions that make difficult moments less likely.

These approaches are especially helpful when you notice patterns, like the same behaviors repeating, certain times of day that are harder, or situations that consistently lead to distress. They're also helpful if you feel like you're always reacting and rarely have a chance to catch your breath.

As with the rest of this book, you don't need to use every strategy here. Read through with curiosity and try what fits your situation right now.

Get Ahead of the Behavior

Many caregivers wait for a behavior to start before responding. That makes sense. We're reacting to what's right in front of us.

But one of the most effective proactive strategies in dementia care is learning how to step in *before* a behavior begins.

Lola cared for her sister, who had Alzheimer's disease. Most evenings, her sister became upset, restless, and anxious. She paced the house, insisted on leaving, and was clearly distressed. After talking through the situation, it became clear that her sister was experiencing sundowning.

Sundowning is a pattern that often shows up in the late afternoon or evening. It can include these responses:

- Increased confusion
- Agitation
- Restlessness
- Anxiety
- Hallucinations
- Irritability or aggression

These symptoms often improve by morning, but tend to return around the same time each day.

In the past, Lola waited until her sister started showing signs of distress and then tried to calm her, distract her, or redirect her. This rarely worked well. By the time the behavior had started, her sister's brain was already overwhelmed, and Lola was left exhausted from trying strategy after strategy with little relief.

Once Lola learned the Get Ahead of the Behavior approach, she made a simple but powerful change: instead of waiting for distress to show up, she paid attention to the pattern.

Like clockwork, her sister's agitation began around 6:00 p.m.

So Lola shifted her support earlier.

Around 5:45 p.m., before the agitation started, she would ask her sister to help her fold towels at the kitchen table. For her sister, folding towels was familiar and calming. For your loved one, it might be something entirely different, and that's okay.

This works because it is much harder for someone to become distressed when they are already engaged and settled. A brain that feels calm and occupied has a better chance of staying that way.

By adjusting *when* she intervened, Lola reduced her sister's sundowning symptoms before they even began.

This did not eliminate sundowning forever. But it made evenings calmer, shorter, and far more manageable for both of them.

We will talk more about choosing effective activities in the next strategy. For now, focus on the timing.

Care in Action: Think about a behavior that happens often.

Does it tend to show up around a certain time of day? Before a specific activity, such as bathing, meals, bedtime, or leaving the house?

Ask yourself:

- *When does this behavior usually start?*
- *What could I do* before *that moment to help my loved one feel more settled?*

Try engaging them in something familiar or comforting *before* the behavior usually appears.

Getting ahead of the behavior won't prevent every difficult moment, but it can reduce how often those moments happen.

Adjust the Activity to Their Ability

One of the hardest parts of dementia is watching someone lose access to the things that once made them feel like themselves.

As dementia affects thinking and processing, activities that once felt easy can become more difficult.

That doesn't mean the activity itself has to be taken away.

If the person still enjoys the activity and it's safe to do so, let them continue to do that activity even if they aren't doing it well (see the "Let Them Do It Wrong (or Differently)" section in Chapter 13).

But what if the person is trying to do an activity that leads them to feeling distressed? Let's say someone who loved doing home projects their entire life is becoming increasingly frustrated when they can't figure out what correct tool they should use for a project. Or, let's say the person who enjoys watching TV can't use the remote without getting frustrated.

These are situations when we want to adjust the activity to their ability.

When we try to stop the person with dementia from engaging in the activity they want, they may begin to see you as the obstacle instead of the ally.

As mentioned in Chapter 2, Mindy's husband had always loved home renovation projects. But as his dementia progressed, his ability to use tools safely became a serious concern. Instead of fixing things, he often broke them further without realizing it.

One day, Mindy found him messing with live electrical wires. She knew she needed to make a change. She also knew that taking it away would feel like taking a piece of him with it.

Mindy found a solution: instead of stopping him from working on projects, she gave him safe items to "fix." She found old, unused objects around the house, such as a VCR, a landline telephone, or a cassette player. She even started visiting thrift stores to find appliances he could "fix" or take apart.

She then asked for his help fixing them, even though they didn't actually need to be fixed.

This helped her husband:

- Continue feeling useful and engaged.
- Experience the joy of working with his hands.
- Stay safe while still doing something meaningful.

Mindy found the right balance. She let her husband participate in something he loved in a way that matched his current abilities and safety needs. She didn't need to explain to him what she was doing. That likely would've upset him. Instead, she just did it.

Adjusting activities is one of the ways we preserve what still brings meaning and joy to our loved ones, even as some abilities become harder for them.

Here are some signs that suggest an activity may need to be adjusted to better match their ability:

- They show frustration because they can't do the task as well as before.
- There are serious safety issues.
- The activity creates significant stress for the caregiver (leading to excessive messes, damage to important possessions, etc.).

Instead of stopping an activity altogether, look for creative ways to adapt it.

> **Care in Action:** Think of an activity your loved one enjoys doing. In what ways could you adapt this activity throughout the course of the disease?

Here are examples of how caregivers have successfully adapted common activities without taking away purpose or enjoyment:

- **They love cooking but struggle with following recipes:** Let them stir ingredients, choose recipes, look through food magazines, taste test, set the table, or help with simpler prep tasks instead.
- **They enjoy gardening but can't manage large tasks:** Provide small potted plants to tend to or let them water flowers with a light watering can or spray bottle, look at videos of gardens, or flip through garden picture books.
- **They love knitting but can no longer follow patterns:** Offer thicker yarn and larger needles for easier handling, encourage them to simply wind yarn into balls, look into no-sew craft projects, introduce other craft projects that don't involve knitting, watch knitting videos, ask them about how they learned to knit, ask them to teach you how to knit.
- **They enjoy painting but struggle with fine details:** Provide larger brushes and simple color-based projects to keep them engaged, introduce finger painting, go to museums and look at paintings, look at their past paintings.

The goal is to preserve their sense of purpose and enjoyment while making the activity accessible and frustration-free.

By adjusting activities to their ability level, you help your loved one stay engaged, feel valued, and experience moments of joy, no matter where they are in their dementia journey.

Limit Advanced Warnings

Carl was caring for his wife, who had dementia. Wanting to help her prepare for daily life, he told her about upcoming appointments, errands, and visits well in advance. He even kept a calendar where he wrote down all upcoming events so she could check it whenever she wanted.

There was just one problem: whenever his wife learned about an event happening later in the day, or even days ahead, she became anxious and started preparing for it immediately.

When she heard about a doctor's appointment two days away, she began getting ready immediately, convinced they needed to leave.

If Carl mentioned a family member was visiting later, she became upset that they hadn't arrived yet and started asking about them repeatedly.

Instead of helping her feel prepared, advanced warnings were increasing her anxiety. She wasn't able to hold onto the idea that the event was happening in the future. Instead, she reacted as if it were supposed to be happening now. Her brain could register the information, but not place it in time.

Carl realized that telling his wife about events ahead of time wasn't helpful. Instead, he started giving notice just before the event happened, or in some cases, not at all. This wasn't avoidance or dishonesty. It was an adjustment based on how her brain was processing information.

Rather than reminding her about an appointment days in advance, he simply said, "It's time to head out," right before they needed to leave.

Rather than telling her about a visit hours ahead of time, he waited until the person arrived and then said, "Look who's here!"

Since she was used to checking the calendar, Carl found another way to use it. Instead of writing down upcoming events, he left sweet messages and reminders of her favorite TV shows. This small shift reduced her stress and made daily life smoother for both of them.

Care in Action: Many caregivers have been told it's best to prepare the person with dementia in advance, but is that working for your loved one? If something creates more stress than relief, it might be time to adjust your approach. Observe how your loved one reacts to advanced warnings:

- Do they become anxious or agitated when told about an upcoming event?
- Do they start preparing immediately, even if it's days away?
- Do they ask repeatedly about the event, unable to hold onto the information?

If so, consider limiting advanced warnings. For many caregivers, this single shift leads to fewer repeated questions, less anxiety, and calmer transitions throughout the day.

Reason from Their Reality

Brenda was caring for her husband, who had dementia. Before his diagnosis, he had owned a successful insurance company, which their son had since taken over.

One night, Brenda woke up to find her husband convinced that a client had broken down on the side of the road and urgently needed their insurance paperwork. No matter what she said, he would not believe her when she told him it was not true.

Desperate to calm him down, she called their son for advice. Her son had taken over the family business years earlier.

Her son had an idea. Instead of trying to convince his father that the situation was not real, he told him that he had already delivered the insurance paperwork to the client and everything was taken care of.

That simple explanation, one that made sense within her husband's reality, instantly calmed him down.

Trying to reason someone with dementia into seeing things your way rarely works. That kind of logic depends on memory and insight that may no longer be available.

But reasoning can work if it makes sense within the person's reality, just as Brenda and her son proved.

The mistake most caregivers make is trying to pull the person with dementia into our reality. That approach often leads to frustration, arguments, and distress.

A helpful way to think about this is to ask yourself:

Would this explanation make sense if I truly believed what they believe right now?

Instead of telling Brenda's husband:

- "You don't work in insurance anymore."
- "There is no stranded driver waiting for paperwork."
- "You are imagining this."

His family entered his reality and said: "The paperwork has already been delivered. The client is all set."

By meeting him where he was mentally, they reassured him without causing more confusion or distress.

This approach is closely tied to the principle of Focus on the Ending, Not Their Understanding. The goal was not to make him understand that he was no longer working. The goal was to help him feel at peace.

For decades, he had been a successful businessman who took pride in taking care of his clients. When caregivers respond in ways that honor a person's long-held identity, the brain often relaxes instead of resisting.

Acknowledging who he had always been, rather than challenging it, made all the difference.

> **Care in Action:** Coming up with responses that make sense within the person with dementia's reality takes practice, but anyone can do it.

Start with one situation where you felt stuck or escalated. Ask yourself, *What explanation would make sense inside their world?* Write down one alternative response you could try next time.

Inside our Care Collective, we once held a session called Creative Responding, when caregivers shared challenging situations they struggled to respond to. Together, we practiced coming up with explanations that fit the reality of the person with dementia.

You can do the same. With practice, this skill becomes easier and more natural, much like building a muscle.

Remove or Replace Triggers

Mandy was caring for her husband, who had dementia. Every time he walked down the hallway and saw a row of family photos, he became visibly upset. These photos had been on the wall for years without issue. Now, for reasons Mandy couldn't immediately understand, they were causing distress.

We often hear that pictures of family members are helpful and calming for people with dementia. That wasn't the case for Mandy's husband. Yet another reminder that there isn't a one-size-fits-all approach to dementia.

Rather than trying to explain who the people in the photos were or correct her husband's reaction, Mandy made a simple change. She removed the photos from the wall. This approach didn't require teaching, convincing, or redirecting. It works because it reduces distress at the source.

With that one adjustment, walking down the hallway was no longer a problem.

Another option could have been to keep the frames but replace the photos with something more neutral, such as nature images. This would have preserved the familiarity of the space while removing the source of distress.

When a trigger can be removed or replaced, it is often one of the easiest and most effective solutions available.

Another common trigger for distress is when items feel lost, stolen, or misplaced.

People with dementia often hide or misplace belongings for a variety of reasons:

- They may believe others are trying to steal from them.
- They may forget where they placed something. Memory changes can make everyday objects seem lost when they were simply set down in an unusual location.
- They may feel embarrassed and want to keep something private rather than ask for help.

When Lee's wife began experiencing urinary incontinence, she started hiding her soiled underwear in unusual places. He found them under furniture, behind houseplants, and even inside her purse. She knew something was wrong and was trying to manage it quietly.

This created a strong odor problem for Lee until he realized what was happening and began checking her usual hiding spots.

Here are some ways caregivers reduce stress around hidden or misplaced items:

- Make copies of important items such as identification cards and keys.
- Store valuable papers and jewelry in a secure location.
- Watch where your loved one goes when they come home, which often reveals consistent drop spots.
- Check the trash before taking it out, since important items sometimes end up there.
- Use small tracking devices on items that frequently go missing and cause distress.
- Regularly check favorite hiding spots.

Your loved one is not trying to create problems. Their behavior is often an attempt to feel safe, private, or in control.

Care in Action: Look around your home and observe where distress seems to start.

Is there a specific object, room, sound, or visual that consistently leads to agitation?

Are there items that are frequently misplaced or hidden in the same locations?

Instead of correcting or confronting the behavior, experiment with removing or replacing the trigger.

Sometimes the most powerful intervention is not what you say or do, but what you quietly change.

Adjust the Environment

Milo cared for his wife, who was in the later stages of Alzheimer's disease. She spent much of her day walking through the house, picking things up and placing them elsewhere. Forks ended up in the bathroom cabinet. The TV remote appeared in a bedroom drawer.

At first, this drove Milo crazy. He was constantly searching for items and growing more frustrated by the day.

Then he had an important realization: instead of fighting a behavior that was not hurting anyone and that actually seemed to keep his wife engaged, he could adjust the environment so it worked better for both of them.

Milo loved spending time in his shed working on projects. He decided to put a lock on the shed door and move anything truly important inside. He stored his wallet, important papers, medications, and even his toothbrush there.

Everything else stayed in the house. If items were moved around, it was no longer a problem.

His wife was able to continue rearranging objects, which clearly gave her a sense of purpose and movement. Milo no longer had to spend his day searching for essentials or correcting a behavior that wasn't dangerous.

His wife never seemed bothered by the locked shed door. If she had been, Milo had other options available. He could have placed a simple "Do Not Enter" sign on the door, covered it with a curtain, or disguised it so it blended into the wall.

Instead of exhausting himself by constantly correcting or redirecting her, Milo made one environmental change that reduced his stress and allowed his wife to continue an activity that brought her comfort.

This approach is not about ignoring safety concerns or allowing harm. If a behavior puts someone at risk, intervention is necessary. But when a behavior is repetitive, non-dangerous, or driven by restlessness or habit, adjusting the environment can be far more effective than trying to stop it.

This strategy works because it shifts the question from "How do I stop this behavior?" to "How can I make this behavior less disruptive?"

> **Care in Action:** Think about a behavior that repeatedly frustrates you or makes daily life harder. Sometimes the most effective solution is not stopping the behavior, but redesigning the space around it. Ask yourself:
>
> - *Is this behavior actually unsafe, or is it just inconvenient?*
> - *Is there something in the environment I could change to make this easier for both of us?*

Wrapping Up: When Prevention Isn't Enough

By now, you have learned how proactive strategies can help prevent many dementia-related behaviors before they start. Small adjustments, such as engaging your loved one before agitation sets in, choosing activities that match their abilities, or removing triggers that cause distress, can make daily life smoother and less stressful for both of you.

But even with the best preparation, some challenges can't be avoided. When behaviors happen despite your best efforts, knowing how to respond in the moment becomes just as important as preventing them.

That's what we'll focus on next.

Chapter 11

In-the-Moment Strategies

No matter how much you plan ahead, there will still be moments in caregiving that catch you off guard. A medication is suddenly refused. Your loved one insists they need to go home, even though they are already there. Or a small moment suddenly turns into something much bigger, and you're left wondering how it got there so quickly.

These situations can feel exhausting and discouraging, especially when it seems like nothing you try makes a difference. They're not a sign that you are doing something wrong. They are part of caring for someone whose brain is changing.

This is where in-the-moment strategies can help. These are responses you can use while something is already unfolding. They are not about fixing dementia or making everything calm. They are about helping you move through a moment without making it harder than it already is.

Let's begin.

Direct Their Attention Where You Want

David was in his late 80s, and his wife, who had dementia, was living in a memory care facility. He spent most of his days visiting her and had slowly put many of his own interests aside.

David loved golf. He had stopped playing years earlier, not because he lost interest, but because golfing upset his wife. Even hearing about it caused distress, so David removed it from his life entirely.

But despite giving up golf, something surprising kept happening.

No matter what David did, when he walked through the door to visit her, his wife would accuse him of golfing instead of being with her. "You were golfing again, weren't you?" she would say.

It did not matter that he had not been golfing.

It did not matter that he had stopped.

Her brain filled in the gap with the same conclusion every time.

David felt stuck. He had already given up something he loved, and now he was still being accused of the very thing he was trying to avoid.

When David joined the Care Collective, we talked through what was actually happening: the problem wasn't golf. The problem was where his wife's attention landed the moment he arrived.

Instead of trying to defend himself, explain, or correct her assumption, David tried something different. He focused on redirecting her attention immediately when he walked through the door.

He began bringing something with him each time he visited that could guide her attention somewhere else right away.

The first time he tried this, he walked in holding a bouquet of flowers.

Much to his amazement, his wife did not accuse him of golfing. Her attention went straight to the flowers. She commented on how pretty they were. They talked about the colors. The accusation never came.

Nothing about her memory had changed. Nothing about her belief system had changed. What changed was the direction of her attention.

The flowers were not the solution. The redirection was.

You don't need to bring flowers. You might redirect attention in other ways:

- A photo to show on your phone
- A story or memory you plan to share
- A small treat or drink to enjoy together
- A simple activity you begin right away

This works because attention is limited. When you intentionally guide it early, there is often less room for assumptions, accusations, or distress to take hold.

Not long after David began using this approach, he sent me a note. For the first time in six years, he had gone golfing again and his wife never even brought up the topic.

> **Care in Action:** Think about a moment when your loved one consistently fixates on the same accusation, worry, or assumption.

Ask yourself, *What could I introduce immediately that might gently pull their attention somewhere else?*

This isn't about avoiding them or giving up more of yourself.

It's about giving the moment a different starting point.

Sometimes, changing where attention lands is enough to change how the entire interaction unfolds.

Redirect After You Show You Care

Redirection is the act of shifting a person's attention from something distressing or unhelpful to something more positive or supportive. It's a common and useful approach in dementia care, especially when a behavior or trigger is escalating.

But redirection doesn't always work. When it backfires, it is usually for one of two reasons.

Reason 1: Redirecting Too Soon

When a behavior shows up that we want to stop, our instinct is often to redirect immediately. We want the behavior to end as quickly as possible.

But when we rush to redirect, we often skip an essential step: connection.

Even if a person with dementia has difficulty understanding words, they can still sense when they are being dismissed. If redirection feels like an attempt to shut them down rather than support them, it often leads to more resistance, frustration, or agitation.

Try connecting before you redirect.

You've likely heard the saying, "The person with dementia is not trying to give you a hard time. They are having a hard time."

Now imagine you are upset about something and the person you are talking to immediately tries to distract you or change the subject without acknowledging how you feel. That would likely feel invalidating and frustrating.

Connection doesn't have to be long or complicated. It can be as simple as:

- Listening to what they are saying.
- Acknowledging their feelings, even if what they are saying is not true.
- Showing interest or concern if they seem upset.
- Briefly joining them in what they are doing before redirecting (see "Join Them Before You Try to Change Them" in the next strategy).

Even one minute of connection can dramatically improve how well redirection works.

Reason 2: The Redirection Is Not Appealing Enough

Another common reason redirection fails is because what we offer in its place is not compelling.

Imagine someone trying to pull you away from something that feels important to you, only to offer something you don't care about. You would likely resist.

For redirection to work, what you are offering needs to be more appealing than what they are currently focused on.

That means:

- Knowing what they enjoy. What foods, activities, objects, or topics reliably hold their attention?
- Planning ahead. Have a few redirection ideas ready before you need them.
- Considering timing. For example, offering coffee might be effective in the morning, but not close to bedtime.
- The better you understand what captures your loved one's interest, the more effective redirection becomes.

> **Care in Action:** Think ahead to moments when you often need to redirect your loved one.

Brainstorm at least four redirection ideas you could try in those situations. Make sure they are things your loved one genuinely enjoys.

When the moment comes: connect first, then redirect.

If something doesn't work, that doesn't mean you failed. It may simply mean the timing, tone, or alternative needs adjusting.

When redirection is paired with connection and something genuinely appealing, it is far more likely to work without resistance or frustration.

Join Them Before You Try to Change Them

Elicia's grandmother had dementia, and every evening she insisted that she needed to go home, even though she was already home. As the evening went on, she would grow anxious, begin packing her belongings, and prepare to leave.

In situations like this, it's natural to try to convince the person with dementia that they are already home. But as you have learned, that approach rarely works.

Many caregivers also jump straight to redirection, quickly trying to shift attention to something else. But when redirection happens too soon, it can feel dismissive rather than supportive.

Instead of rushing to change the behavior, joining first can build trust and emotional safety. That connection often makes redirection possible later.

Some caregivers worry that joining a behavior will make it worse. In reality, it is often the attempt to stop or correct the behavior too quickly that increases distress. You know your loved one best, so use your judgment, but do not be afraid to try this approach when it is safe.

Rather than arguing with her grandmother or trying to convince her she was already home, Elicia decided to join her.

She helped her grandmother pack. She wrapped a few small items and placed them into a box as if they were preparing to leave together.

After a few minutes, her grandmother became calmer. She felt supported and reassured because her family was helping her.

That's when Elicia suggested taking a short break for coffee and a snack.

While they were eating, the box was quietly put away. The next evening, when the same concern came up, the process was repeated.

Because Elicia joined her grandmother first, her grandmother felt heard and supported. Only after that connection was established was redirection successful.

Joining does not mean agreeing with something that is untrue. It means entering their experience long enough to reduce fear and build trust. Joining them shows you care about their experience, which naturally helps them relax.

> **Care in Action:** If it is safe to do so, the next time your loved one starts doing something you want to change, pause before correcting or redirecting.

Ask yourself these questions:

- *Can I join them for a moment before trying to change this?*
- *What would it look like to show support first?*

Even joining for one minute can lower tension and make the rest of the interaction smoother.

When someone feels you are on their side, they are far more likely to move with you instead of against you.

Highlight the Undesirable Consequences

I hesitated to include this strategy. It's not a first-line approach, and it is not appropriate for everyday use. When used carelessly, it can create unnecessary distress or damage trust.

However, when used thoughtfully and sparingly, this strategy can be effective in situations when something truly important needs to happen and other approaches have failed.

This approach works by gently highlighting a real, meaningful downside of not taking action. It's not about threatening, scaring, or shaming the person with dementia. It's about helping their brain weigh a consequence that still makes sense to them.

The key is this: the consequence must align with the person's long-standing values or priorities, not with fear.

Here is an example that illustrates this well.

One caregiver was struggling to get her mother bathed. Her mother had not bathed in months and insisted she had already done so, even when she had not. Gentle reminders, reassurance, redirection, and making the bath more appealing had all failed.

This was becoming a serious hygiene and health concern.

The caregiver knew something important about her mother. She had grown up during the Great Depression and had always been deeply uncomfortable with waste, especially wasting water, food, or electricity.

Instead of arguing about whether her mother had already bathed, the daughter tried a different approach.

She filled the bathtub with warm water and then said calmly, "I just filled this tub, but I guess I will have to waste all this water."

Her mother immediately looked uncomfortable. Wasting water did not sit right with her.

The daughter then added, "Or we could just make good use of it now, and then you won't have to bathe tomorrow."

Her mother agreed to the bath.

Nothing about this approach involved fear. There was no arguing. No correcting. No pressure. The daughter simply highlighted an outcome that mattered to her mother and framed the bath as the more comfortable option.

This worked because it aligned with who her mother had always been.

Important guidelines for using this approach:

- Use it only when the situation truly matters, such as hygiene, medical care, or safety.
- Make sure the consequence is real and meaningful to the person, not exaggerated or frightening.
- Keep the explanation brief and calm. One or two sentences is enough.
- Watch their response closely. If it increases anxiety, guilt, or shame, stop using this approach.

This strategy should never feel threatening. If it does, it is not the right fit.

Care in Action: Think about a situation when your loved one is refusing something important and other strategies have not worked.

Ask yourself these questions:

- *Is this an issue with real consequences for their health or safety?*
- *Is there a value, belief, or lifelong priority that still matters to them?*
- *Can I frame the situation in a way that feels collaborative rather than corrective?*

This is not a strategy for everyday use. But in specific situations, when used with care and respect, highlighting an undesirable consequence can help move things forward.

Overlook Their Objections

Niko has dementia and does not like taking a shower. Whenever his wife tells him it is time to bathe, he insists that he has already showered.

It would be easy to correct him, argue, or try to convince him otherwise. But doing that only reinforces his objection and keeps the focus on resistance.

Instead, his wife chooses not to engage with the objection. When Niko says, "I already showered," she calmly replies, "Okay. That's fine. I have this one ready for you, too."

Then she gently leads him toward the shower and continues with her plan. She hears what he says, but she does not dwell on it or try to prove him wrong. Her attention stays on the goal of getting him bathed rather than on winning the argument.

This approach works for several reasons:

- It avoids reinforcing the objection. The more attention we give to resistance, the stronger it often becomes. By not arguing or correcting, the objection does not become the center of the interaction.
- It keeps momentum moving forward. Instead of getting stuck in back-and-forth resistance, the interaction continues calmly toward the intended outcome.
- It reduces pressure. Simply acknowledging what they say without debating it can make it easier for them to follow along.

Overlooking objections doesn't mean ignoring distress or forcing activity. If someone becomes frightened, agitated, or unsafe, this approach should stop. But when the objection is repetitive, habitual, or rooted in memory loss rather than true refusal, this strategy can prevent unnecessary struggle.

> **Care in Action:** Is there a task your loved one regularly resists, such as bathing, eating, or getting dressed?

Instead of arguing or correcting, try acknowledging their response and gently continuing toward the goal. Notice whether keeping the interaction moving forward reduces resistance or emotional intensity.

Similar to the Do Less to De-Escalate strategy in Chapter 10, there are moments when the most effective response is not engaging with the objection at all.

Make It Enticing

Joanne was caring for her mother with dementia. She and her husband had planned a much-needed vacation for respite, but there was a problem. Her mother didn't want to stay with her son while Joanne was away.

Two weeks before the trip, Joanne joined one of our live calls feeling defeated. She was considering canceling the vacation and trying to get a partial travel refund while there was still time.

As we talked, it became clear why her mother was refusing.

Joanne had explained that her mom needed to stay with her son so she could be supervised while Joanne was gone. Her mother did not believe she needed supervision and insisted she would be fine staying home alone.

Most adults don't like the idea of being watched or supervised. It feels restrictive and unnecessary. So instead of focusing on why her mother needed to go, we shifted to a different question: why would she want to go?

I asked Joanne what her mother loved most about her son's house. Her answer was immediate: her grandchildren. Joanne's mom adored spending time with them, and they adored her. That was our opening.

Instead of framing the stay as something necessary for her safety, Joanne reframed it in a way that felt inviting. She told her mom that her grandchildren had been working on special art projects just for her.

Now staying at her son's house was not about being supervised. It was about spending time with her grandchildren.

Her mom happily agreed to go.

Making something enticing can completely change how a person responds. Instead of focusing on what they have to do, shift the focus to something they want to do.

It doesn't have to be big. Even small motivators can make a difference.

When you want your loved one with dementia to do something, look for a way to make it enticing to them. This is a simple but powerful strategy that is often overlooked.

Care in Action: Think of something you want your loved one with dementia to do. Reconsider how you are describing it.

Is there a positive or meaningful reason they might want to do it?

The more appealing something feels, the more likely they are to cooperate without resistance or frustration.

Use Flattery

Tiffany's mom frequently misplaced items and became frustrated when she could not find them. Instead of assuming something was misplaced, she often blamed Tiffany: "What did you do with my purse?"

It would have been easy for Tiffany to defend herself, but arguing would only have escalated the tension. Instead, she tried a different approach: "Gosh, I've never been as organized as you. How did you get to be so good at keeping everything in order?"

Rather than pushing back, Tiffany used flattery to shift the tone of the moment. Her mom's anger softened almost immediately, and the conflict dissolved.

Instead of fueling frustration, Tiffany's response highlighted her mother's strengths. That shift helped her mom feel admired instead of upset.

Flattery often works because of the following reasons:

- It redirects frustration without argument. Compliments change the emotional direction of the moment rather than escalating it.
- It taps into preserved identity. Many people with dementia still take pride in certain qualities, such as being organized, intelligent, capable, or dependable.
- It creates an emotional reset. Positive emotions can interrupt agitation and make cooperation more likely.

Tiffany eventually began keeping a small notebook of the responses she used with her mom and noted which ones worked best. Over time, she learned which compliments were most effective and leaned on those consistently.

You can do the same.

Flattery works best when it is grounded in something that is true about them. It is not about being sarcastic or manipulative. It is about speaking in a way that helps them feel respected and settled in the moment.

> **Care in Action:** Think of a recent situation where your loved one became upset with you.

Ask yourself these questions:

- *What strength or identity could I have highlighted instead of defending myself?*
- *What compliments are most meaningful to them based on who they have always been?*

The next time tension builds, try using a sincere compliment and observe how it changes the interaction.

Tap into Positive Memories

Ray's wife rarely wanted to shower or bathe. Each time he tried, she responded with "I already bathed," even though it had been months since she had stepped into the shower.

Ray tried everything:

- Calling it a "spa day" to make it sound luxurious.
- Reasoning with her, even pointing out that she smelled.
- Keeping a shower calendar to show her the last time she bathed.

Nothing worked.

Then one day, Ray tried something different. Instead of telling her to shower, he used a phrase she had often said herself before dementia was ever in the picture.

For much of their marriage, when they had plans to go out, his wife would tell him she was going upstairs to "get pretty." That was her way of saying she's on her way to get ready for the date.

One day, he told her to "go upstairs and get pretty."

To his surprise, she did exactly that. She went into the bathroom, showered, got dressed, and "got pretty."

For his wife, that phrase tapped into something familiar and positive. It connected to a time when she took pride in her appearance and enjoyed getting ready. It felt natural, not corrective or demanding.

At the time Ray shared this success, his wife had willingly showered and "gotten pretty" for three straight weeks.

Ray reached his goal of improving his wife's hygiene without pressure, embarrassment, or resistance.

The key takeaway is this: you don't always have to name the task you want your loved one to do. Instead, tie the task to a familiar phrase, routine, or memory that feels meaningful and exciting to them.

This works because long-held emotional and procedural memories often remain accessible even when short-term memory and reasoning do not.

Procedural memory is the part of the brain that remembers how to do things that were repeated over many years, like getting dressed, setting the table, or following familiar routines. Even when facts are forgotten, these patterns can still guide behavior.

For example:

Medication time: "Let's have our afternoon tea and cookies."

Bedtime: "It's story time."

Exercise: "Let's pump you up!" (said in an Arnold Schwarzenegger voice)

The goal is to match the wording to their personality and life history, then experiment until something clicks.

> **Care in Action:** Think about your loved one's past routines, sayings, and habits. What phrases did they use repeatedly? What activities once brought pride, comfort, or enjoyment?

Try reframing a difficult task using language that feels familiar and positive. Experiment gently and observe what works.

Sometimes, the right words make all the difference.

We'll explore this more in Chapter 12.

Repeat What Works

When caring for someone with dementia, you might find yourself responding to the same behavior over and over. Just like having the same conversation multiple times, your loved one may repeatedly experience distress about the same issue, whether it's believing something that isn't true, waking up scared, or feeling confused in a familiar situation.

Diana cared for her husband, who had dementia. Many mornings, he would wake up terrified, feeling as if he were falling. Each time, she would take his hand, reassure him that she was there, and tell him everything was okay. Within moments, he would calm down and recognize that he wasn't falling. This happened several times a week.

It's easy to assume that if a behavior keeps happening, your response isn't good enough. Many caregivers tell me, "I tried that, but the behavior keeps happening."

But if your response helps calm and comfort your loved one in the moment, then it *is* working. The fact that the behavior happens again doesn't mean your approach needs to change. It simply means you need to keep using the same response. You don't need to reinvent your response every time.

When you find something that soothes or reassures your loved one, repeat it. Consistency can be comforting, and using a familiar approach can help them settle more quickly.

Care in Action: If a behavior keeps happening, remind yourself that it's okay to respond the same way each time, especially if it brings comfort. The behavior happening again isn't a sign that your approach isn't working. It's a sign to keep using that approach!

Wrapping Up: Responding with Confidence in the Moment

It's impossible to know the perfect response to every difficult situation. No single strategy will work every time. Dementia care requires flexibility and a willingness to try different approaches depending on the day, the situation, and the person in front of you. Some responses may work well for a while and then stop working. As the dementia changes, what works will change, too.

These in-the-moment strategies can help you move through difficult situations when tensions are especially high.

As you move forward, pay attention to what seems to help your loved one settle, feel safer, or recover more quickly. Those responses are worth repeating.

In Chapter 12, we'll shift our focus to communication strategies. These tools will help you think about how words, tone, and timing can reduce resistance and make everyday interactions feel more cooperative and less draining.

You can move on when you feel ready.

Chapter 12

Communication Strategies: How to Speak in a Way That Works

Dementia changes how a person understands and how they express themselves. That means you might be saying something clearly, but their brain isn't taking it in the same way. Or they may know what to say, but can't get the words out.

This makes it frustrating for everyone involved.

Family members often struggle to say things in a way their loved one can understand, while the person with dementia is struggling to be understood.

When language changes become more noticeable, they may be described as *aphasia*, a condition many people with dementia develop that affects speaking, understanding words, reading, or writing. This helps explain why conversations that once felt easy or enjoyable can start to feel stressful or exhausting. But even without a formal diagnosis like aphasia, communication can still become difficult in many different ways.

Sometimes it can feel like you're speaking a language you aren't fluent in.

This chapter is about helping those moments feel more workable. You will learn practical ways to adjust how you speak, listen, and respond so communication feels less strained and more supportive.

Choose Your Words Wisely

I once worked with a man whose daughter was juggling a full-time job and many other responsibilities. Her father loved being active and social, but she didn't have the time to engage with him as much as he wanted.

She hoped he would attend a nearby adult day care center to give him opportunities to socialize and stay active. But as soon as he heard the term *day care*, he didn't like the idea. After all, he was a grown man, why would he need day care?

In talking to his daughter, we talked about what he really enjoyed and what mattered to him. She told me he was a smart man who always loved school and learning. Using that information, we introduced the idea again. But this time, we called it *school*. We talked about how he would be able to meet other students and learn new things. That small shift in language changed everything.

From then on, one of my favorite times to visit this client was right after he got back from "school." He would walk in with a smile on his face and a piece of paper in his hand, usually some sort of worksheet or "assignment" he had completed at the day center.

I saw the power of language again with another caregiver in my Care Collective program. Her father lived with her, but she needed extra help so she could continue working.

He didn't like the idea of having someone come in to "watch" him, insisting that he didn't need supervision.

Instead of calling the home health aide a caregiver, we referred to her as his "assistant." As a retired dentist, he was used to always having an assistant in his office. That simple adjustment allowed him to accept help easily because, in his mind, he was simply working with an assistant again.

Language matters. The words we use can shape how a situation feels.

Notice the difference in the following words. What do you think your loved one would respond to best?

- Facility versus community
- Shake versus smoothie
- Medication versus vitamins
- Home health aide versus friend
- Diapers versus underwear

There is no right or wrong choice. It's about finding what resonates with them. The name doesn't have to make sense to anyone else. It only needs to be something that feels comfortable and familiar to your loved one. If calling medication *vitamins* makes it easier for them to take, then that's the right word to use. However, someone who is highly focused on their health might prefer the term *medication* because they want to follow their doctor's recommendations closely.

If calling an adult day program *school* helps them engage, then that's what matters. You can even make up a word that only the two of you know! It doesn't have to make sense to anyone else—just something your loved one accepts.

> **Care in Action:** Take a moment to reflect on the words you use with your loved one. Are there certain words that seem to trigger a negative response? Could you reframe them in a way that feels more natural or positive? Experiment with different terms and observe what works best.

A small change in language can make a big difference in cooperation, comfort, and connection.

Practice the Art of Conversation

Most conversations follow a familiar rhythm. Someone asks a question, and we answer it. Someone makes a statement, and we respond.

With dementia, that rhythm can break down quickly, especially when a question leads to confusion, accusations, or distress.

Caregivers often tell me, "I answered honestly and somehow everything spiraled."

Here's an example of how easily that can happen: imagine a person with dementia has created a piece of artwork and enjoys showing it to family members. The family has already seen the same artwork several times that day.

Person with dementia:	"Did you see my artwork?"
Caregiver:	"Yes, it was lovely."
Person with dementia:	"Who showed it to you? People are always taking my things!"

The caregiver answered truthfully, but the conversation took an unexpected and upsetting turn.

This is where logic starts to work against you.

Now look at a different response.

Person with dementia:	"Did you see my artwork?"
Caregiver:	"No."
Person with dementia:	"It was here earlier. How come you missed it? Did someone take it?"

Even though the answer changed, the outcome did not.

This is what I call the *yes or no trap.*

When someone with dementia asks a question, answering directly can unintentionally pull the conversation into confusion, suspicion, or frustration. Not because you said the wrong thing, but because their brain may not be able to track the logic or timing behind the answer.

In moments like this, a simple and effective response is to keep the conversation open by saying something like "Tell me about that."

Let's try it in the same scenario:

Person with dementia:	"Did you see my artwork?"
Caregiver:	"Tell me about that."
Person with dementia:	"I painted a tree today."
Caregiver:	"That sounds lovely. You're such a good painter."

You don't always need to answer the question. You just need to keep the conversation going.

Instead of getting stuck in a yes or no response, this approach keeps the conversation moving forward. It enables the person with dementia to share what matters to them, without putting pressure on memory, logic, or accuracy.

This works because questions in dementia are not always about getting factual answers. Sometimes they are about connection, reassurance, or engagement. A direct answer can unintentionally create confusion if it doesn't match what they expect or remember.

By responding with an open invitation instead, you avoid asking their brain to solve a problem it can no longer reliably manage. You shift the focus away from facts and toward connection.

Care in Action: The next time your loved one asks a question or makes a statement and you are unsure how to respond, try saying, "Tell me about that."

Notice how it changes the direction of the conversation.

Keeping the conversation open can reduce resistance, prevent unnecessary conflict, and help your loved one feel heard and valued, without requiring you to correct, explain, or defend.

Don't Highlight Their Need for Help

The way you offer help matters just as much as the words you use. When help feels like it's pointing out what they can't do, it often leads to resistance. If they don't believe they need help, pointing out their limitations often backfires. The goal is to offer it in a way that doesn't feel like help at all.

Lila's husband was no longer safe staying home alone. Before heading to an appointment, she told him that someone would be coming over to "watch him" while she was gone. Her husband became upset, stormed off, and even threatened to harm the helper.

Later, Lila realized why he reacted so strongly. He did not feel supported. He felt supervised.

The next time Lila needed to leave, she took a different approach. Her daughter-in-law, who lived nearby, had offered to help whenever needed. But rather than telling her husband that someone was coming to watch him, Lila came up with a better plan: she told him that their daughter-in-law was having Wi-Fi issues at her house and needed to come over to use their internet.

Now, instead of feeling like he was being supervised, he felt like he was helping someone else and Lila was able to leave, knowing he was safe.

The help didn't change. The story did.

This shows up in other situations, too.

I was explaining the approach at one of my speaking engagements and a woman in the audience shared how her husband sometimes got stains on his shirt but resisted changing into a clean one. Instead of pointing out the stains and making him feel self-conscious, she simply offers him a backrub. No mention of the stain. No pressure to change.

When he agrees, she helps him take off his shirt, gives a short backrub, and then hands him a fresh, clean shirt when they are done. No argument, no resistance. Just a smooth transition.

We don't always need to explain why we're doing something, especially if it highlights what they can't do.

Simple ways to reduce struggle without pointing out difficulty:

- If they need help cutting food, serve it precut.
- If they spill drinks often, use cups with lids.
- If they struggle with the remote, replace it with a simpler one.

Care in Action: Think of something your loved one struggles with but doesn't want help for. How could you offer support in a way that preserves dignity rather than highlights difficulty? Look for small adjustments that make the task easier without calling attention to what they can't do. Even small changes can make daily life smoother for both of you.

Be Mindful of How You Look

Most people with dementia experience slower processing speed, meaning it takes longer for them to think, understand, and respond. As language becomes harder to follow, they often rely more heavily on nonverbal cues, such as facial expressions, tone of voice, posture, and movement.

This means how you look and carry yourself can matter just as much as, and sometimes more than, the words you use.

Even if your words are calm and kind, a tense face, rushed movements, or hesitant body language can communicate stress or uncertainty. Your loved one may respond to that stress, even if they can't explain why.

Think of yourself as a mirror. Your expression, tone, and body language help signal to the person with dementia how safe or stressful a moment is.

There is a brain-based reason for this. Our nervous systems are wired to pick up on the emotional states of people around us—this happens automatically, below conscious awareness. When someone sees tension or frustration on another person's face, their own nervous system often responds in kind. When they see calm, confidence, and warmth, their brain is more likely to settle.

This effect becomes even more important in dementia, when reasoning and language are less reliable, but emotional processing remains strong.

Consider a common caregiving moment, like helping your loved one take a shower. You might choose your words carefully and speak in a gentle tone. But if your face shows hesitation because you are bracing for resistance, your loved one may sense that uncertainty and become anxious or resistant as well.

I know this can be hard, especially when you are tired, overwhelmed, or stressed. It's not about being perfect or hiding how you feel. It's about recognizing that small, intentional shifts in your physical presence can help your loved one feel safer and more at ease.

A relaxed expression, open posture, calm movements, and warm eye contact can communicate reassurance before a single word is spoken.

Care in Action: The next time you interact with your loved one, pause for a moment and check in with yourself.

If you could see yourself in a mirror, what would your face and body be communicating? Do you look rushed, tense, or braced for conflict? What small shift could you make to appear calmer, more open, or more confident?

Even subtle changes in how you carry yourself can influence how your loved one feels and responds in the moment.

Spark Conversations

Many caregivers tell me they struggle with knowing what to say to their loved ones. They feel like they're having the same conversations over and over, and those conversations can feel repetitive, dull, or short-lived.

Before we dive into ways to spark engaging conversations, it's important to recognize that your experience of the conversation and your loved one's experience may be completely different.

For a person with dementia, each time they share a story might feel like the first time. They may genuinely enjoy the conversation, even if you've heard it a hundred times. If they're engaged, smiling, or content, the conversation is serving its purpose even if it's repetitive. We don't need to change anything.

The other thing to think about is the goal you have for the conversation. If your goal is to have deep, meaningful discussions, you may find yourself feeling disappointed or frustrated. But if your goal is to create moments of connection and social interaction, you may find it easier to embrace these conversations even if you'd had them many times before.

Conversation isn't about new information. It's about shared experience.

If you want to spark new conversations, try focusing on older, pleasant memories. Choose topics that connect to long-term memory and ask open-ended questions that invite them to share.

Memories from earlier in life, and the emotions tied to them often stay with a person even when recent memories are harder to remember.

For example, if your loved one enjoys music, you might ask questions like these:

- Who is your favorite band?
- What's your favorite song?
- Tell me about your favorite concerts?
- Who did you go to concerts with?

To encourage childhood memories, you could ask questions like these:

- How did you spend the holidays growing up?
- What was your favorite part of school?
- Did you go on any family vacations?
- What was your first job?

Simply asking about positive memories can open up conversation, create moments of joy, and help you learn new things about your loved one. This approach is often used in dementia care and is sometimes called *reminiscence therapy*.

Some people with dementia may have a harder time responding with words. That can make the conversation feel one-sided, but it doesn't mean connection isn't happening. Sharing a memory of your own, like a funny childhood story or a favorite vacation moment, can still create connection. You may notice signs they're engaged, like smiling, nodding, or making eye contact. Even without words, they can still enjoy the moment.

Care in Action: Choose a topic your loved one is likely to enjoy and ask a few open-ended questions. You don't need their answers to be accurate or complete. The goal isn't to exchange information, it's to create connection.

If the conversation becomes one-sided or your loved one struggles to respond, you can keep sharing in a calm, natural way and notice signs of connection, like smiling, eye contact, or relaxed body language. Even when words are limited, shared moments of connection still matter.

Be Active in Your Listening

When someone with dementia is trying to communicate, their words may not come out clearly or make sense. But how you respond still matters.

Listening in a way that shows you're paying attention helps your loved one feel heard, and respected, even when you don't fully understand what they're saying. This alone can ease frustration and build trust.

Active listening doesn't mean understanding every word. It's about showing presence, interest, and care.

Here are ways to practice active listening:

- Give your full attention. Put away distractions, turn toward them, and keep gentle eye contact.
- Use nonverbal cues. Nod, smile, or lean in slightly to show engagement.
- Reflect what you hear. Try responses like, "It sounds like that meant a lot to you" or "It seems like you're feeling frustrated."
- Encourage them to continue. Simple phrases such as "Tell me more" or "That sounds interesting" invite connection.
- Be patient. Allow extra time for processing and responding without rushing or finishing their sentences.
- Avoid correcting. If something is inaccurate, focus on the emotion behind what they are saying rather than the facts.

At times, your loved one may mumble, mix up words, or speak in ways that are hard to follow. They may not realize this is happening. Even in those moments, how you respond still matters.

If you don't fully understand what they're saying, you can stay engaged by nodding, smiling, keeping a relaxed posture, and using simple affirmations like "Oh really?" or "I see."

You don't have to understand every word for someone to feel heard.

Care in Action: The next time your loved one is talking, focus less on understanding every detail and more on how you are showing that you are listening. Notice your eye contact, body language, and tone. Respond with patience and curiosity rather than correction.

Wrapping Up: Communication That Connects

By now, you've seen that communication with someone who has dementia goes far beyond words. It's about connection and meeting them where they are. Small shifts, like adjusting your language, listening more closely, or being mindful of your facial expressions and body language, can help lower frustration and strengthen your bond.

There's no single right way to communicate, and what works one day may not work the next. Even the same approach can land differently depending on the person and the moment.

Some people with dementia may feel frustrated if you finish their sentence when they are taking a long time. Others may feel relieved that they don't have to keep struggling to find the words. The key is to watch how your loved one responds and adjust.

If communication is becoming more difficult, some families also find it helpful to work with a speech-language pathologist for additional support and ideas.

As you keeping going, remember that your words, tone, and presence shape how your loved one experiences the moment. Keep practicing these strategies, trust what you are noticing, and give yourself grace. Dementia care can often feel difficult, and every effort you make to communicate with patience and care matters.

The goal isn't perfectly balanced conversations. It's meaningful moments of connection.

In Chapter 13, we'll look at how support needs change over time and how you can continue showing up as the disease progresses.

Chapter 13

Strategies for Adapting to Their Reality

Dementia changes how your loved one experiences the world.

What feels obvious or familiar to you may no longer make sense to them. What worked yesterday may stop working today. When that happens, trying to hold on to old expectations, routines, or logic often leads to more frustration for everyone involved.

This chapter is about what it means to stop fighting that shift.

Adapting to their reality doesn't mean giving up or pretending things aren't hard. It means responding to what is actually in front of you, rather than what you wish were different. When you adjust your approach to match where their brain is now, moments can feel less tense and more workable.

With these strategies, you'll learn how to loosen the need for correction, stay flexible when things are done differently or imperfectly, and move with the moment instead of against it. These shifts aren't about lowering standards. They're about staying connected as dementia changes the rules, even when that means letting go of how things used to be.

Let Them Do It Wrong (or Differently)

As dementia changes, your loved one may struggle with activities they've always enjoyed. You can adjust the activity to match their ability, but sometimes it helps to let them do it their way, even if it's not done the "right" way.

Take Donna's story, for example. She recently joined the Care Collective and shared that every morning for the past 30 years, her husband read the *Wall Street Journal.* Lately, though, when she asked him what he read, he couldn't recall details or he mixed up the facts.

She worried this meant it was time to take the newspaper away and find a new activity for him. But he showed little interest in anything else.

I asked her two simple questions:

- Did her husband seem upset while reading?
- Did he seem bothered that he couldn't remember the details?

She said no to both.

That's when things became clear: it wasn't her husband who was struggling. It was Donna.

Her husband was perfectly happy reading the paper, even if he was no longer fully understanding the information. The problem wasn't the activity. The problem was how painful it was for Donna to watch his decline.

In this situation, there was nothing to fix. He wasn't frustrated. He wasn't distressed. The routine still brought him comfort, and that mattered more than whether he fully understood what he was reading.

This is an important shift in caregiving. Not everything that looks "wrong" needs to be corrected. It's okay if they read without understanding.

It's okay if they cannot remember details.

It wouldn't even matter if they held the paper upside down.

As long as the person with dementia is engaged, content, and safe, sometimes the best thing you can do is let them be.

Care in Action: The next time your loved one is doing something "wrong," pause and ask yourself these questions:

- *Are they safe?*
- *Are they upset or distressed?*

If the answer is no, it might just be that it's hard for you to watch. If they are content and not in danger, resist the urge to correct them.

This also applies to words and beliefs. Not every incorrect statement needs to be corrected. Dementia caregiving comes with many real challenges. Harmless mistakes don't need to be one of them.

Let Them Say It Wrong

People with dementia will naturally get facts wrong. They may believe things that aren't true or recall details incorrectly. This is common, and in most cases, you don't need to do anything at all. You can simply let it go.

Every time we correct our loved one, we put an unnecessary strain on the relationship. Over time, even if they can't remember exactly why, they may start to associate us with someone who makes them feel bad. That makes it harder for them to trust us when they do need help.

It's okay if they remember things incorrectly. The question isn't whether something is factually correct. The question is whether correcting it serves any meaningful purpose.

If you're concerned about them sharing misinformation with others, you can decide whether it's necessary to privately give the correct information to the other person without noticeably correcting your loved one.

For example, I remember interviewing a patient in his 70s while his adult daughter sat beside him. As part of the assessment, I asked about his alcohol use.

Proudly, he told me he drank six beers a day.

Surprised, I repeated the amount back to him for confirmation. He nodded. Six beers a day.

His daughter sat quietly, listening. She didn't say a word.

Later, she called my office. Her dad was drinking six non-alcoholic beers a day, and he didn't know they were non-alcoholic. She didn't want to embarrass him or cause an argument, so she chose not to correct him in the moment.

This was a perfect example of when it mattered for me to have the correct information, but correcting him would've made things worse.

In many cases, it's not even necessary to privately give the correct information. Sometimes, the best thing you can do is simply let them say it wrong and move about your day.

Care in Action: The next time your loved one says something incorrect, ask yourself these questions:

- *Is it absolutely necessary that I correct them?*
- *Would correcting them create more stress or frustration?*
- *Can I just let it go?*
- *Who benefits if I correct this?*

By choosing when to correct and when to let things be, you'll reduce conflict, build trust, and create more positive interactions.

Remember the Power of Presence

People with dementia experience sadness, frustration, and emotional pain just like the rest of us. But as caregivers, we often feel a strong urge to fix things when our loved one is upset. But not every moment needs to be fixed.

Imagine one of your closest friends, someone without dementia, is sad because a loved one no longer calls or visits. They feel abandoned, and their heart hurts.

> How would you respond? Would you immediately change the subject?
>
> Would you try to distract them?

Probably not. That would feel dismissive and insensitive. Instead, you would likely sit with them, listen, and offer comfort, knowing you can't fix the situation.

Now think about how we often respond when someone with dementia expresses sadness.

- We might correct them: "They did visit last week. Do you not remember?"
- We might minimize their feelings: "Oh, don't worry. I'm sure they are just busy."
- We might redirect them before they have had a chance to process their emotions: "Look what's on TV. Let's watch."

But people with dementia are still people. Their emotions are real, even if their memory of events is not. The pain they feel in that moment is still real.

If their feelings make sense based on what they believe is happening, being with them is often more helpful than trying to fix it.

Rather than rushing to fix or redirect their sadness, try being with them, just as you would with anyone you care about. Your presence alone can be deeply comforting.

Let them talk.

Acknowledge their feelings.

Sit beside them or offer a gentle touch.

In moments like these, you don't have to take the pain away. Just being there with them matters.

> **Care in Action:** The next time your loved one feels sad or frustrated, resist the urge to fix the situation. Instead, be present with them, just as you would with a close friend. Listen, acknowledge their feelings, and give them space to feel what they're feeling. It's not easy to sit with that, but being there with them often matters more than anything you could say or do.

Go with the Flow

Just like not every emotion needs to be fixed, not every behavior needs to be corrected. Sometimes, the easiest, least stressful approach is to let things be.

One Careblazer shared a story about her husband, who believed people were watching their home and planning to break in when they left.

Each time they got in the car and backed out of the driveway, he would duck down in the passenger seat, trying to make it look like someone was still inside. He stayed that way until they were out of the neighborhood.

In his mind, so long as the other people thought someone was in the home, they wouldn't break in.

Rather than trying to convince him that no one was watching the house, she let him do what helped him feel safe. Within a few moments, he would sit back up, and things would settle.

Nothing dangerous was happening. No harm was being done. But arguing or correcting him would've created fear and resistance where none needed to exist.

By going with the flow, she avoided an unnecessary struggle and kept the peace.

> **Care in Action:** Think about a situation where your loved one's behavior isn't harming them but goes against what makes sense to you. Instead of correcting or reasoning with them, try going with the flow and see if it allows the moment to pass more easily. You might be surprised at how much smoother things feel when you don't try to correct everything and just let them be.

Enjoying Nonperfect Moments

Toward the end of my mom's life, she needed a walker. There was just one problem: she didn't want to use it.

Every time I visited, I'd find it in the same exact spot, untouched. Meanwhile, she shuffled her feet along the tile floor in house slippers, something that would make any physical therapist break into a cold sweat. She was a walking fall risk, and the hard tile floor wouldn't be forgiving if she ever lost her balance.

At first, I spent most of my visits trying to convince her to use the walker.

I explained the risks. I made logical arguments. I even tried to make the walker more appealing. Nothing worked.

And the worst part? I was wasting my precious time with her arguing instead of enjoying the moments we had left.

I finally realized something: I didn't want to spend every visit fighting about a walker.

Of course, I still wanted her to use it. But I also wanted to enjoy my time with her. I was letting one less-than-ideal situation take over everything, when in reality, pushing and pressuring her was only making her more resistant.

So I backed off. I realized that insisting on the walker was costing me the very thing I wanted most, feeling connected to her.

I didn't stop caring. I didn't stop hoping she'd eventually use the walker. I just stopped letting my frustration over what wasn't working ruin the time when we were together.

The truth is, we can keep working toward a goal (like getting a loved one to use a walker) while also accepting the reality of the present moment.

When I stopped pushing, I was able to relax. We had better visits. And, ironically, by taking the pressure off, I found myself in a better place to come up with creative solutions instead of just repeating what wasn't working.

This isn't giving up. It's simply letting go of an approach that reality has shown doesn't work. Safety still mattered. I simply stopped letting one unresolved issue ruin every visit.

Care in Action: What is one area where your loved one seems to resist care? How are you handling it right now? What would happen if you let go of the pressure for just one interaction and focused only on enjoying your time together?

Try it. You might be surprised by how much lighter everything feels.

Make Light of the Heavy

I have a brilliant and beautiful friend named Nicki whose father had Lewy body dementia, which causes visual hallucinations. When he was alive, he often saw "tree people" outside their living room. He believed there were men standing near the trees in their yard.

Nicki, who also happens to be extremely witty and single, didn't panic or try to argue when he talked about the "tree people." Instead, she quipped, "Are any of them single?"

Her dad laughed, and just like that, the conversation moved on. Humor helped his nervous system settle without challenging his reality.

Nicki and her family understood that these hallucinations were a regular part of his condition. Correcting him would not help, because what he was seeing felt real to him. Instead of arguing or escalating the moment, she used humor to help both of them move on.

Rather than correcting him or turning it into a serious issue, she found a way to bring lightness to the moment, making it easier for both of them to move on.

Humor can be especially powerful when it turns moments of embarrassment or discomfort into shared humanity.

At one of my keynote presentations, I was sharing about how powerful humor can be in caregiving. A member in the audience raised her hand. She shared that her husband with dementia also has urinary incontinence and she helps him change his disposable briefs throughout the day.

Then she said something that had the entire room burst into laughter: "When it's time for him to change, I tell him it's time to pull out the 'astronaut underwear!'"

Every time, this makes both of them smile, turning what could be an uncomfortable or frustrating moment into a shared joke.

Caregiving is filled with serious and heavy moments, but that doesn't mean we can't find joy and humor along the way.

Of course, humor works best when used sensitively and in a way that fits your loved one's personality and the situation. Some people respond well to lightheartedness, while others may feel dismissed or embarrassed by it. The key is to gauge their reaction and use humor as a way to connect, not dismiss or make fun of their feelings.

> **Care in Action:** Think about a situation in your day that feels especially heavy or tense. Ask yourself whether a playful phrase, nickname, or shared joke might soften the moment. This could be something silly, familiar, or meaningful only to the two of you. Try it once and notice their reaction. If it brings ease or connection, keep it. If it doesn't, let it go.

Whose Perspective Are You Considering?

I once worked with a caregiver who had recently moved her mom into a care facility. Wanting to preserve a sense of normalcy, she continued a long-standing tradition. Every Wednesday, she picked her mom up and took her out to her favorite lunch spot, something her mom had done for years.

At first, this felt like the loving thing to do.

But over time, June noticed something troubling. Whenever her mom left the facility, she became anxious. She hesitated to get into the car. When it was time to return, she resisted getting out. The anxiety wasn't subtle. It was consistent.

Still, June kept the routine going. She told herself, "This is what mom would have wanted."

Her mom, however, was communicating something different. At the facility, she was calm. She participated in activities. There were no signs of agitation. The anxiety only appeared when she left and when she returned.

June was viewing the situation through her own perspective. She understood the history of the tradition. She understood its meaning. From her point of view, continuing the lunches felt kind and respectful.

But from her mom's perspective, leaving the facility each week was stressful. Returning was even worse.

Once we shifted the lens, a new option became clear. Instead of taking her mom out, June began bringing her mom's favorite lunch to her room. They ate together there, without the anxiety of transitions. The tradition remained, but it was adapted to match her mom's current needs.

Dementia changes many things, including traditions we've held for years.

It can also change what we make behaviors mean.

Recently, I spoke with a caregiver who was overwhelmed with guilt because every time she called her mom, her mom asked, "When can I come home?" Each time she heard that question, it felt like a knife to the heart.

But as she talked more, an important detail emerged. During in-person visits, her mom never asked about going home. Staff at the facility reported that she was settled, calm, and at ease in her environment.

The distress appeared only during phone calls.

In this case, the phone call itself seemed to be the trigger. Hearing her daughter's voice may have activated memories of "home," even though her day-to-day experience at the facility was peaceful.

The caregiver had options. She could continue calling and work on how she responded to the question. Or she could reduce how often she called, knowing it increased her mom's anxiety. Most likely, she would do a combination of both.

The key shift was this: the question "When can I come home?" wasn't necessarily a sign of suffering. It was a response to a specific trigger, the phone call.

In dementia care, behaviors are information. Before reacting, it helps to pause and ask yourself, *Whose perspective am I using to interpret this moment?*

What feels loving or logical to you may not feel that way to your loved one. When you see it from their side, it often becomes easier to see what might actually help.

Sometimes what's painful isn't the behavior or the situation, but the story we're telling ourselves about what it means.

Care in Action: When a behavior feels confusing or upsetting, pause and ask yourself these questions:

- *What might this situation feel like from their perspective?*
- *When does this behavior happen, and when does it not?*
- *Is this activity serving them, or is it serving my expectations, habits, or guilt?*

Small adjustments can reduce anxiety significantly, especially when we let the person with dementia's experience guide our decisions.

Let Their Response Guide You

When caregivers ask me whether a certain strategy is "right" or "wrong," my answer is often the same: look at how your loved one responds.

Dementia care can't be judged from the outside. A strategy that looks helpful to one person may feel confusing or distressing to another. What matters is not how the strategy looks, but how it is experienced by the person with dementia.

For example, some caregivers wonder about offering a baby doll or a stuffed animal. From the outside, people debate whether this is comforting or demeaning. But that debate misses the most important question.

How does the person with dementia respond?

Some people may feel offended, upset, or anxious. They may feel burdened by what feels like a new responsibility. For them, this approach increases distress and is not helpful.

Others, often in more advanced stages, may experience comfort, joy, and a sense of purpose. They may become calmer, more settled, and more emotionally regulated. For them, the same approach is deeply soothing.

The strategy itself is not the problem.

The response tells you everything you need to know.

You can't judge a dementia care strategy on the surface. You can only judge it based on its impact. In general, approaches that reduce distress, increase calm, or bring comfort are worth continuing. Approaches that increase agitation, fear, or resistance are signals to try something different.

This doesn't mean you will get it right every time. It means you are paying attention to the most reliable guide available to you: the person in front of you.

Care in Action: When trying a new approach, ask yourself these questions:

- *Does this reduce distress or increase it?*
- *Do they seem calmer, safer, or more settled afterward?*
- *Or do they seem more anxious, upset, or resistant?*

Let their response guide your next step. There is no universal "right" strategy. There is only what helps this person, in this moment.

Wrapping Up: Embracing Their Changing Reality

Caring for someone with dementia means constantly adjusting, not just to their needs, but to how they experience the world. It requires flexibility, patience, and a willingness to let go of expectations that no longer serve them or you.

Adapting to their reality often means letting go of how things used to be and responding to what helps right now. When you do that, interactions tend to feel calmer and less threatening for your loved one.

These strategies are about meeting them where they are and letting go of unnecessary battles so you can focus on what truly matters: connection, comfort, and quality time together.

Chapter 14

Rethink Failure

We've just covered a wide range of dementia caregiving strategies. And chances are, you're going to try one of them and it won't work.

That's because caregiving doesn't follow a book. It follows real life.

Every day, things like how your loved one (or you) slept, what your loved one ate, who is around, the time of day, and countless other factors can influence how a situation unfolds. The same strategy that worked yesterday may fall flat today.

Allow yourself not to know.

Allow things to feel unclear, confusing, or imperfect.

One of the most helpful mindsets a dementia caregiver can adopt is a scientist's mindset.

Scientists don't expect to be right all the time. In fact, much of science moves forward because researchers discover that what they once believed to be true is incomplete, inaccurate, or no longer applies. Ideas evolve. Understanding changes. New information replaces old assumptions.

A good scientist is not attached to being right. They're attached to learning. They experiment.

They observe. They stay curious. And they are comfortable saying, "I don't know yet."

That same mindset is incredibly useful in dementia care.

What works beautifully today may not work tomorrow. A response that calms your loved one this week might do nothing next week. A strategy that helps in the morning may fail completely in the evening. That doesn't mean you did something wrong. It means the situation changed.

Caregiving is not about finding the one perfect response and repeating it forever. It is about noticing patterns, trying approaches, observing reactions, and adjusting as the disease progresses.

When you take a scientist's approach, a "failed" strategy is no longer a failure. It becomes information.

You learn that:

- Timing mattered.
- Tone mattered.
- The environment mattered.
- Your loved one's needs shifted.

Instead of thinking, *I handled that wrong,* you can begin asking these questions:

- *What did I notice?*
- *What changed?*
- *What might I try differently next time?*

This mindset also takes pressure off you as a caregiver. You are not expected to have all the answers. Even the most brilliant scientists do not. They stay open to being surprised.

A scientist doesn't argue with data. They get curious about it.

That curiosity is powerful in dementia care, especially when your loved one says something that isn't true or reacts in a way that doesn't make sense to you. You don't have to agree with what they are saying. You don't have to correct them. You don't have to argue.

Instead, you can approach the moment with curiosity:

- *What might this feel like for them?*
- *What emotion could be underneath this?*
- *What are they trying to solve or communicate?*

When you respond to the experience your loved one is having rather than trying to stop or fix it, their guard often comes down. You are not lying. You are not giving up. You are acknowledging how their world feels to them right now.

Adopting a scientist's mindset helps you to stay flexible, compassionate, and open as dementia changes the rules again and again.

You're not failing when things stop working. You are learning. And that learning is one of the most important caregiving skills of all.

You don't have to analyze every moment.

There will be days when you don't want to evaluate, adjust, or try a new strategy. Days when the only goal is to get through. That is valid. It is respectful toward yourself.

You're allowed to take mental breaks. Not every challenging moment needs to become a learning lesson.

Part III

The Support: Focusing on the Caregiver

Chapter 15

Your Emotional Toolkit

"Everyone keeps saying to take care of yourself, but no one tells you how you are supposed to do that!"

Even the best caregiving strategies stop working when you're depleted.

You don't need to become more patient or more positive. You need something that actually helps when you're tired and still have to keep going.

Well-meaning people often tell caregivers, "Take care of yourself" or "You deserve a break." I'm sure they're trying to be helpful when saying these things, but for many caregivers those words can actually feel frustrating.

You're already doing everything you can just to get through the day—Managing behaviors, appointments, medications, safety concerns, and emotional landmines.

Being told to "take care of yourself" can feel like another item on a never-ending to-do list. It can feel like a luxury rather than a necessity. Never mind the part where no one tells the caregiver how to actually do that in a way that's possible.

This section isn't about bubble baths, morning routines, or adding more tasks to your already full plate.

It is about helping you get through this without burning out.

Even with the best information and the best caregiving strategies, it's incredibly hard to respond well when you're overwhelmed.

Many caregivers already know what might help. The problem isn't a lack of knowledge. The problem is capacity.

When you're exhausted, patience is thinner. Creativity is harder to access. Small decisions feel heavy. Even strategies that worked yesterday can feel impossible today.

That's why caregiver strategies matter just as much as behavior strategies.

There's a growing push to make the world more dementia-friendly. That's great. But a dementia-friendly world is not possible without caregiver-friendly support.

Caregivers are the ones holding everything together. If you are exhausted, overwhelmed, and unsupported, no amount of dementia-friendly language or programs will be enough.

Burnout doesn't happen because you're doing something wrong. It happens because the demands are relentless, the stakes are high, and the support is often inadequate.

Self-care, in this context, is not indulgence.

It is not optional.

And it is not selfish.

It is about protecting your physical health, your emotional well-being, and your ability to keep showing up over time.

Just as you've learned to adjust expectations for your loved one with dementia, this section invites you to adjust expectations for yourself.

You will learn practical strategies that reduce strain, conserve energy, and help prevent crises before they happen. These are not about doing more. They are about doing things differently.

Some of these strategies may feel uncomfortable at first. Letting go of certain standards. Asking for help earlier than feels necessary.

Accepting that being a good caregiver does not mean being endlessly patient, cheerful, or self-sacrificing.

That discomfort is part of change.

Caregiving is not a sprint. It is a long, unpredictable journey.

This chapter, and those that follow, are for you.

Nicety Versus Necessity

As caregivers, we often hold ourselves to a very specific standard of what "good care" should look like:

- Home-cooked meals.
- Daily baths.
- Tidy houses.
- Clean clothes.

Those standards might make sense when life is stable and energy is plentiful. But dementia caregiving rarely offers either.

One caregiver in our community once described this as "suspending the healthy people routine."

In other words, letting go of expectations that made sense before dementia, but no longer fit the reality you're living in.

As dementia changes their routines, it often means we have to change ours, too.

There will be days when you are utterly exhausted. Those are not the days to cook a 45-minute meal or insist on a perfectly coordinated outfit. Those may be the days for takeout, cereal for dinner, or letting your loved one wear the same shirt three days in a row without turning it into a battle.

You may notice resistance as you read this. Many caregivers carry a strong internal image of what "great care" looks like. The truth is, you can't sustain that level of care when you are completely depleted.

Sometimes, adjusting what is acceptable is exactly what allows you to keep going. This is where the filter of necessity versus nicety becomes especially helpful. When stress is high, letting go of some niceties is not a failure. It is a survival strategy.

Necessities are the things that must be done. Safety. Food. Basic hygiene.

Niceties are things that are nice, but not required.

A spotless house.

Perfect meals.

Daily showers no matter what.

You might not want cereal for dinner every night, but on a particularly hard day, it may be the kindest option for both of you. You may prefer a tidy home, but during overwhelming weeks, it's okay if the laundry sits on the couch a little longer.

This is not about lowering your standards permanently. You can always choose differently tomorrow.

Think about a time before you were caregiving when you were exhausted or burned out. You likely cut corners, rested more, and gave yourself grace. That same compassion applies here.

Choosing necessity over nicety is not *bad* care. It is *realistic* care. And it's what helps you to keep showing up, day after day, year after year.

Care in Action: Take a moment to reflect on today.

Ask yourself these questions:

- *What feels absolutely necessary right now?*
- *What feels nice, but not essential?*

Now ask one more question:

- *If I were not worried about what anyone else might think, what is one thing I could let go of today?*

Choose one nicety you can release without compromising safety. For example:

- Order takeout instead of cooking.
- Skip a nonessential task.
- Let an outfit, a meal, or a routine be "good enough."
- Choose rest over perfection.

Notice what happens when you make that choice.

Do you feel a little less pressure?

A little more space to breathe?

You can always revisit your standards tomorrow. Today, give yourself permission to choose sustainability over appearances.

Make Things Simpler When You Can

Reducing stress as a dementia caregiver doesn't always mean reducing caregiving tasks.

Often, it means reducing *life* tasks.

When I was in the thick of caring for my parents, I remember one moment clearly. I had just washed the sheets and duvet cover and was standing in the bedroom, struggling once again to wrestle the duvet into its cover. I felt irrationally angry. Exhausted. Completely over it.

And in that moment, I decided I was done with duvets. I replaced them with quilts. Bed-making instantly became easier. Faster. Less frustrating. That decision had nothing to do with dementia care. But it made a meaningful difference every single weekend after laundry.

Caregiving already asks so much of you. If everyday life is unnecessarily complicated on top of that, stress builds quickly. Simplifying where you can is not laziness. It's strategy.

Small changes in your environment and routines can free up more energy than you might expect. Take a moment to ask yourself: *What do I do regularly that could be replaced, removed, or outsourced?*

Here are some caregiver-friendly ways to simplify life:

- **Cut laundry stress:** Instead of lots of outfits, stick with a smaller rotation of easy-care clothing. Darker colors or patterns hide spills better and reduce pressure for constant washing.
- **Duplicate essentials:** Keep multiple sets of frequently used items, such as glasses, phone chargers, nail clippers, and slippers, in different rooms. Fewer searches mean fewer interruptions and less frustration.
- **Minimize decision fatigue:** Rotate the same five to seven familiar meals your loved one enjoys. Grocery shopping becomes predictable, meals require less thought, and you avoid the daily decision of "What's for dinner?"
- **Outsource the little stuff:** If it is an option for you, consider outsourcing repetitive tasks. This might mean grocery pickup or delivery, mailed medications, laundry services, or occasional housecleaning. This is not available to everyone, but for some

caregivers, it can meaningfully reduce mental and physical strain when resources allow.

- **Reduce the daily reports:** Many caregivers feel obligated to constantly update family members. These well-meaning check-ins can become draining. Consider setting limits or using a shared document for major updates so conversations don't revolve entirely around caregiving.

Remember: Simplifying your life does not mean you care less. It means you are protecting your energy for what truly matters. When caregiving is already complex, your life doesn't also need to be.

Care in Action: Choose one small part of your daily routine that feels more draining than it needs to be. Ask yourself these questions:

- *Does this truly need to be done this way?*
- *Could it be simplified, reduced, duplicated, or done less often?*
- *Is there one small change that would save me time or energy this week?*

Start with just one adjustment. You don't have to overhaul your life or change everything at once. This is about noticing where friction exists and gently removing it.

Reducing effort in one area often frees up energy for what matters most.

Your Goal Isn't to Make Them Happy All the Time

Previously, we talked about paying attention to how the person with dementia responds as a way to guide our approach. That can be incredibly helpful. But, like most things in dementia caregiving, it is not always that simple.

Here is the important caveat: no matter how skilled, thoughtful, or compassionate you are, there will be times when the person with dementia becomes upset or unhappy because of something you said or did.

That does not mean you did something wrong.

Trying to keep your loved one with dementia happy most of the time may sound like a worthy goal, but it's not possible. Nor is it safe.

In fact, one of the hardest requirements of being a good caregiver is doing things your loved one may not like, but that are in their best interest.

Because dementia affects insight and judgment, many people no longer understand their own limitations. The person may want to drive, live alone, eat spoiled food, or give money to a virtual stranger they believe loves them. From their perspective, these desires feel reasonable. From yours, they are dangerous.

One of your core responsibilities as a caregiver is to keep your loved one safe, even when they do not understand why. If they fully understood the risks, they would not be in these situations to begin with.

That means there will be moments when your loved one is angry with you, frustrated, or unhappy about a decision you made. They may not like what you are doing. They may not agree with you. And that still doesn't mean you are doing anything wrong.

This is one of the most emotionally difficult parts of caregiving. You are asked to act in your loved one's best interest even when they cannot see it and cannot thank you for it.

Of course, we can often reduce distress by using the communication and behavior strategies you have already learned, such as not highlighting their need for help. But no strategy will eliminate every hard moment.

When these situations arise, it is important to remind yourself of this truth: keeping someone safe sometimes means being the person they are upset with.

Your goal isn't to make your loved one happy all the time. And your goal isn't to make yourself happy all the time either.

Sometimes the goal is safety. Sometimes it is stability. Sometimes it is simply getting through the day with the least harm possible.

That, too, is good caregiving.

> **Care in Action:** Notice how often guilt shows up automatically when your loved one is unhappy. Gently challenge that reflex and remind yourself that being a good caregiver doesn't mean avoiding distress at all times. Sometimes it means making thoughtful decisions, even when they are hard and your loved one doesn't understand.

Sometimes the most compassionate choice is also the most uncomfortable one.

Talk to Yourself Like You're Someone You Actually Care About

As a dementia caregiver, there is a good chance you have experienced guilt. Maybe even shame. You may replay moments in your head when you lost patience, said the wrong thing, or wished you could escape for a while. And then you judge yourself harshly for it.

Caregivers are often their own worst critics. That inner voice can be relentless. And it's not harmless.

When you are constantly criticizing yourself, your body stays on high alert. Stress builds. Exhaustion deepens. It becomes harder to recover emotionally, even on days when nothing especially bad happens. In other words, how you talk to yourself matters.

What I often notice is this: the things caregivers say to themselves privately are things they would never say out loud to another human being, especially someone they love.

If someone you cared about lost their patience one day, would you tell them they should feel ashamed? If they needed a break, would you accuse them of being selfish? If they made a mistake, would you tell them they were failing?

Most caregivers would never speak that way to someone else. Yet many do exactly that to themselves, dozens of times a day.

This kind of inner dialogue slowly drains your emotional fuel. It eats away at confidence, compassion, and motivation. And it makes an already difficult role even heavier.

Talking to yourself with care does not mean ignoring mistakes or pretending caregiving is easy. It means responding to yourself the way you would respond to someone you genuinely care about. With understanding. With perspective. With humanity.

You are allowed to be human in this role.

Care in Action: Pay attention to how you speak to yourself in the quiet of your own mind. When you notice harsh or critical self-talk, pause and ask yourself, *What would I say to someone I love in this situation?* Then practice saying that to yourself instead.

This is not indulgence. It's self-preservation. And it is one of the most powerful ways to protect your ability to keep going.

Asking for and Accepting More Help

If there is one thing most dementia caregivers deserve, it is more help.

The demands of caregiving are relentless, and doing everything alone is not sustainable.

When caregivers talk to me about help, I hear the same concerns over and over again.

- "No one is willing to help."
- "People say they'll help, but they don't follow through."
- "I don't even know what to ask for."
- "My loved one only wants help from me."

Underneath all of that is often a quieter belief: *I should be able to handle this.*

Here is something important to hear clearly. You do not have to *need* help in order to accept help. You do not have to wait for things to get "bad enough."

Many caregivers delay asking for help until exhaustion, resentment, or health problems force the issue. But waiting for a crisis is one of the hardest and most stressful ways to get support. When we are overwhelmed, we often accept whatever solution appears first, even if it is not what we would have chosen under calmer circumstances.

The truth is that every caregiver will need help in one way or another. No single person can do this alone, not if they want to keep their loved one safe, and not if they want to protect their own health. Wanting help is reason enough to receive it. You do not have to justify it by reaching a breaking point.

A helpful place to start is simple awareness. For a few days, notice everything you do that doesn't actually require your physical presence. This is not yet about what you want help with. It is about noticing how much you carry.

Many daily tasks fall into this category: cooking, grocery shopping, cleaning, laundry, yard work, running errands, picking up prescriptions, or sitting with your loved one for short periods of time.

That list becomes your list of possible support.

Just because something *can* be delegated does not mean it *should* be. If grocery shopping is your one escape out of the house, you may want to keep it. If cooking brings you comfort, you may want to continue doing that. Help should make your life easier, not take away the few things that still give you a sense of normalcy.

Once you have a sense of what could be shared, choose just one task that would be nice to get help with. It doesn't have to feel urgent. It just needs to feel helpful. Then choose one person or service you could ask.

This is the part that feels uncomfortable, probably because asking for help is unfamiliar. Be specific:

- "Would you be willing to pick up groceries once a week?"
- "Could you sit with her for an hour on Tuesdays?"
- "Would you be able to help with yard work twice a month?"

If the answer is no, you are not worse off than before you asked. You just have more information. Asking for help is a skill, and like any skill, it becomes easier with practice.

If making a direct ask feels too hard right now, keep your list in mind for moments when people offer help. Many caregivers freeze when someone says, "Let me know if there's anything I can do," not because they don't want help, but because they don't know how to translate that offer into something specific.

The next time you hear that phrase, try responding with, "You know, I've actually been looking for help with ______" or "Do you happen to know anyone who could help with ______?"

Most people want to help. They just don't know what would actually be useful.

Another way support can show up is by letting trusted people know what's going on. One caregiver I worked with lived in the same neighborhood for decades. It was not until late in her husband's illness that she told her neighbors what was happening. She did so initially for safety reasons, in case he wandered. What surprised her was how that honesty opened doors. Neighbors checked in. Help appeared. One neighbor happened to be a nurse and became an unexpected source of support when her husband needed catheter changes.

Another caregiver shared her situation with the community pickleball group she belonged to. Without even asking, the group encouraged her to leave early instead of staying to help with cleanup after activities.

People can't respond to what they don't know.

And if a small voice inside you resists accepting help, remember this: there's no extra recognition for doing this alone. There's a cost to your body, your health, and your ability to keep going.

> **Care in Action:** This week, do one small thing. Write down three tasks that don't require your physical presence. Choose one task that would be nice to get help with. Identify one person or service you could ask. Practice making a clear, specific request.

Remember, relief is not something you have to earn.

Stop Comparing Your Caregiving

"I don't have it that bad." I hear this phrase all the time from caregivers.

It often comes up when someone is considering asking for help, bringing up a concern, or admitting they are struggling. They hesitate. They minimize. They stop themselves.

They might say it out loud, or they might just think it quietly and move on.

Sometimes this belief comes from listening to other caregivers who are further along in the journey. You hear stories about loved ones who no longer recognize family members, who wander, who need full-time care. And suddenly, your own struggles feel small by comparison.

Maybe your loved one repeats the same questions.

Maybe they want to watch the same TV program all day.

Maybe they are still physically independent, but emotionally exhausting.

Maybe things feel hard, but not "hard enough."

So you tell yourself:

- I shouldn't complain.
- I shouldn't need help yet.
- I should be able to handle this.

But caregiving is not a comparison game.

There is no scoreboard. There is no threshold you have to cross before your experience counts.

There is no prize for waiting until things get worse.

Different does not mean easier.

Your caregiving situation may look different from someone else's, but that doesn't mean it's less stressful. It doesn't mean it takes less emotional energy. And it doesn't mean you are less deserving of support.

When caregivers compare themselves to others, they often silence themselves. They push down questions. They delay asking for help. They dismiss early signs of burnout.

And when we deny ourselves support, even for what seem like small things, we lose opportunities to feel better, to adjust sooner, and to prevent unnecessary suffering.

Caregiving is not meant to be endured quietly.

Remember:

- Your experience matters now, just as it is. Not only after it gets worse.
- You don't need a dramatic crisis to justify feeling overwhelmed.
- You don't need to wait until you are falling apart to ask for help.
- You don't need to prove that you have it "bad enough."

When you measure your pain against someone else's, it often keeps you stuck.

When you take your own experience seriously, things can start to shift.

You ask for help sooner. You adjust earlier. And you don't have to carry it alone for as long.

Care in Action: Notice when the thought *I don't have it that bad* shows up.

When it does, pause and ask yourself these questions:

- *Would I say this to another caregiver in my situation?*
- *What support might help me right now, even if things are not at their worst?*
- *What would change if I stopped judging my experience to others?*

You do not have to wait for things to get worse before you deserve support.

Your caregiving experience matters exactly as it is. Even if it's different from someone else's.

Create a Safety Net

"There's no one else who can help."

Many caregivers believe this, and for some, it feels painfully true. They are the default caregiver. The organizer. The safety net. The only one who truly knows what needs to be done.

But here is a question worth asking, even if it feels uncomfortable: "What would happen to your loved one if something happened to you?"

There was a widely reported news story about actor Gene Hackman, who had Alzheimer's disease and was being cared for by his wife. When his wife unexpectedly died at home, Gene was left alone for days without anyone realizing what had happened. By the time authorities were alerted, both had passed.

That story made headlines because of who he was. But this kind of situation isn't rare.

Many caregivers have no backup plan in place. Not because they don't care, but because thinking about it feels overwhelming, frightening, or unnecessary. Some believe they don't have anyone to ask. Others assume they will "figure it out later."

The truth is, creating a safety net doesn't require a perfect plan, major sacrifices, or someone who lives nearby.

It requires one trusted person and a simple agreement.

Think of someone you trust. This could be a friend, family member, neighbor, church member, or even someone who lives in another state.

Create a plan where you check in with them every day. This can be as simple as a thumbs-up emoji, a short text, or a quick call. The content does not matter. The consistency does.

If they don't hear from you on a given day, they reach out. If they cannot get in touch with you, they follow the instructions you have agreed on in advance.

Those instructions might include the following:

- Whom to call locally.
- Whether to request a welfare check.
- How to access key information about your loved one.

This is not a plan you hope to use. It's a plan you hope you never need.

But having it in place provides something invaluable: peace of mind.

Creating a safety net is one of the quietest and most loving forms of caregiving.

Care in Action: You are not planning for disaster.
You are planning for safety. And that is an act of care.

- Choose one trusted person.
- Decide on a simple daily check-in method.
- Agree on what they should do if they cannot reach you.
- Write down essential information such as medications, doctors, and emergency contacts, and let your backup person know where to find it.

Allow Yourself to Have (and Not Have to Explain) Limits

Many caregivers feel as though everyone has an opinion about how they should be caregiving. Family members question decisions. Friends suggest what they would do differently. Some people openly tell you they think you are doing something wrong.

When you are already carrying the weight of constant decisions, safety concerns, and uncertainty, this outside input can be exhausting. Especially because most caregivers are already second-guessing themselves. Caregiving requires so many judgment calls, and the person you are caring for often can't guide or reassure you.

This is where limits matter.

Not everyone will agree with your decisions. Some people will be uncomfortable with the choices you make. That doesn't mean you are doing anything wrong.

Your role is not to manage everyone else's comfort or approval. Your role is to keep yourself and your loved one as safe, supported, and steady as possible.

When limits are not protected, caregiving conversations can quietly turn into long explanations. You may find yourself justifying decisions over and over, answering the same questions, or bracing for criticism every time the phone rings.

That constant explaining drains energy you do not have to spare.

Setting limits is not about controlling other people. It is about deciding what *you* will do to protect your capacity.

Sometimes that means making a clear request.

"I know you mean well, but hearing suggestions about how I should be doing this is not helpful for me. I'm making the best decisions I can with my loved one's healthcare team."

And sometimes it means deciding what you will do if the pattern continues.

"If this continues, I won't be able to take these calls."

Notice the focus:

You are not demanding that someone change.

You are calmly stating what you will do to take care of yourself.

Limits don't have to be harsh. They don't have to be dramatic. And they don't have to be explained repeatedly.

Many situations don't require firm boundaries at all. But when a behavior is repeated and consistently adds strain to your caregiving, you are allowed to respond:

- You are allowed to answer fewer calls.
- You are allowed to change the subject.
- You are allowed to stop explaining your decisions.

You don't owe anyone an ongoing justification for protecting your capacity.

Caregiving already asks so much of you. You are allowed to decide where your energy goes.

Care in Action: Pay attention this week to where you feel pressured to explain or defend your caregiving decisions.

Ask yourself these questions:

- *Whom do I feel obligated to justify myself to?*
- *What conversations leave me feeling drained afterward?*

Choose one small way to protect your energy. That might mean making a simple request, shortening a conversation, or deciding not to engage at all.

Setting limits does not make you unkind. It's what helps you keep going.

Protect What's Yours

I once worked with a man who was caring for his wife with dementia. She loved rummaging through drawers, closets, and every room of the house. Nothing was off limits, including his personal belongings.

Over time, he began to feel as though nothing was his anymore. Eventually, he started carrying his toothbrush with him everywhere, just so it would stay clean, safe, and where he could find it.

When you are caring for someone with dementia, it can start to feel as though your entire world revolves around them. Your routines change. Your space changes. Even your belongings no longer feel secure. It can feel as though your life has been slowly overtaken, and that your own needs, preferences, and boundaries no longer matter.

That loss is not small.

When caregivers have no protected space, no sense of ownership or privacy, stress increases. Resentment builds. And many caregivers begin to feel invisible in their own homes.

Reclaiming something that is just yours is not selfish. It helps you keep your footing.

Another Careblazer I worked with decided to make his garage his sanctuary. He kept the door locked and protected that space for himself alone. Inside, he worked with tools, called friends, and sometimes simply sat and cried. That space gave him somewhere to exist as himself, not just as a caregiver.

This doesn't have to be a room. It can be a drawer, a shelf, a closet, a chair, or a corner of the house. What matters is that it is yours. Protected. Untouched.

Having something that belongs only to you is a reminder that you still exist as a person, not just as a role.

> **Care in Action:** Consider what you could protect just for yourself.

Ask:

- *Is there a small space I could designate as mine?*
- *Is there something I could keep safe that does not need to be shared or managed?*
- *What would help me feel less erased in my own home?*

Choose one small thing and protect it intentionally.

Don't Let Every Decision Feel Like a Test You Could Fail

There are so many decisions families make for a loved one with dementia. In the earlier stages of the disease, those decisions are often made together, with the person with dementia contributing and sharing their wishes. As the disease progresses, that becomes harder.

In the middle and later stages, the person may no longer fully understand the decision or everything it involves.

This leaves many caregivers feeling anxious about making the "right" choice and terrified of making the "wrong" one.

This strategy isn't about choosing perfectly. It's about how you carry decisions after they're made.

Many caregivers get stuck in a mental spiral long before a decision is even made. They replay options, imagine worst-case outcomes, and try to predict the future. The decision may still be undecided, but the emotional toll has already begun.

And even after a decision is made, the doubt often doesn't stop.

In this section, I want to help you think through major caregiving decisions in a way that reduces unnecessary self-blame and prevents you from getting trapped in a cycle of regret and second-guessing.

Amy was caring for her mom at home. Over time, her mom needed more hands-on help with basic tasks. Getting out of bed and moving safely around the apartment became increasingly dangerous. She was falling more often, growing weaker, and needed supervision throughout the day.

Amy was doing everything she could to keep her mom safe. But she was one person. Finding consistent help was difficult. If the home health aide didn't show up and Amy needed to run an errand, she was faced with an impossible choice: leave her mom alone in a situation that was no longer safe, or cancel everything else in her life.

After a lot of thought, Amy decided to move her mom into a nearby care facility.

Two weeks later, her mom fell and broke her hip. When Amy told me this, she said, "I made the wrong decision."

I didn't agree.

I asked her why she made the decision to move her mom into the facility in the first place. She immediately talked about the increasing fall risk, her mom's weakness, and the toll the situation was taking on her own physical health as the only consistent caregiver.

Then I asked her a key question: "Do you like your reason for making that decision?"

She said yes.

That question matters more than almost any other when making major caregiving decisions.

Liking your reason doesn't mean other people have to like it. And it doesn't mean the decision feels good. Most caregiving decisions are painful. It means the reason makes sense to you, given your values, your limits, and the situation you were facing at the time.

If Amy had said, "Because people kept telling me I should" or "Because I felt judged," those would be reasons worth reconsidering. But her reason was safety, what she could realistically manage, and her own physical limits. That mattered. She could stand behind her reason.

Then we talked about the fall.

Amy believed that because her mom fell shortly after the move, the move itself must have been the wrong decision. In her mind, she assumed the fall wouldn't have happened if her mom had stayed at home.

I asked her how she knew that. She didn't.

This is something our brains do under stress. When an outcome is painful, the mind creates an alternate story where a different decision would have led to a better result. But because that version of events never happened, there is no way to know if it would have been better.

Her mom could have fallen at home. The injury could have been worse. She could have been alone on the floor while Amy was out running errands instead of receiving immediate medical attention.

When you catch yourself thinking, *If only I had chosen differently*, be careful. Because when we imagine an alternate outcome, we almost always imagine a better one. We forget that it could just as easily have been worse.

In real time, we cannot predict the future. All we can do is make decisions with the information we have and choose reasons we can stand behind. That's what protects you later.

When doubt shows up, as it almost always does, you don't need to relive the decision or punish yourself. You remind yourself why you made it. You anchor back to the reason, not the outcome.

These are big decisions. Feeling nervous or uncertain doesn't mean you made a mistake. It means you're human.

Sometimes, the support we wish we had from others is the support we need to offer ourselves. The same steadiness. The same compassion. The same reminder that we did the best we could with what we knew at the time.

Care in Action: When doubt shows up after a major caregiving decision, pause.

Doubt is not proof that you made the wrong choice.

Bring your attention back to **why you made the decision in the first place.**

Remind yourself of those reasons.

If something difficult happens after your decision, be careful not to treat the outcome as evidence that the decision itself was wrong. You don't actually know what would have happened if you had chosen differently. Things might have been better. They also might have been worse.

When your mind starts doubting, remind yourself, *I made the best decision I could with the information I had at the time.*

Wrapping Up: Caring for the Life You're Living

Notice something about the strategies in this section:

- None of them require more hours in the day.
- None of them require expensive resources.
- And none of them ask you to become a different kind of person.

That matters, because one of the biggest reasons caregivers struggle with the idea of self-care is the belief that it requires time or money they simply do not have.

These strategies are not about adding more to your plate.

They are about making small but meaningful shifts in how you think, how you respond, and how you use the energy you already expend every day.

They are designed to make caregiving more livable.

Of course, it would be ideal if our healthcare systems, workplaces, and communities automatically wrapped caregivers in support. Many do not. That reality is unfair. And it's not your fault.

But these strategies are here because they are within your control.

You are the one holding this book.

You are the one making dozens of decisions every day.

And even small shifts, practiced consistently, can change how heavy this role feels.

You do not need to implement everything at once.

In fact, I recommend you do not.

Choose one strategy.

Try it for a week.

Notice what changes, not just in what you do, but in how you feel.

I've never been particularly fond of the term *self-care*.

It implies something separate. Something indulgent. Something "extra."

What you are doing here is not that.

Everything you do to protect your energy, your health, and your emotional capacity directly benefits the person you are caring for.

This is not self-care. It is life care. It is caring for your life and your loved one's life at the same time. Because it is impossible to give what you do not have. And it is impossible to offer steady, compassionate care when you are overwhelmed and depleted.

These strategies are meant to help you keep going. But even when you do everything "right," there is still something we need to talk about.

We've talked about caregiving strategies. Now it's time to talk about caregiving realities. The realities that make all these strategies feel overwhelming and sometimes impossible to try.

Because dementia caregiving hurts.

And no amount of strategy can remove that entirely.

That's where we go next.

Chapter 16

Managing a Grief That Doesn't End

This chapter is here to name what many caregivers feel but rarely have words for, so that you don't mistake pain for personal failure.

One caregiver I worked with met a friend for coffee for the first time in what felt like years. As she sat there, she was struck by something she wasn't expecting.

"There was so much living happening," she told me.

People were talking. Laughing. Walking past the window. Making plans. Having conversations about ordinary things. It felt almost shocking to witness.

She realized how small her world had become.

Caregiving has a way of doing that. Slowly, quietly, your life begins to narrow. Your routines change. Your home changes. Even your sense of what is normal begins to shift. Bedrooms start to look like hospital rooms. Calendars empty out. Conversations revolve around medications, appointments, and safety.

Many caregivers have told me some version of the same thing:

"I forgot that this isn't normal."

"I feel like I'm living at the end of a rope."

This disorientation is what happens when caregiving becomes the center of your life.

Dementia itself adds another layer of grief because it is never still. Your loved one may struggle deeply one day and seem almost like themselves the next. A strategy that works beautifully today may fail completely tomorrow. Just when it feels like you've found your footing, a new symptom appears and you are back at square one.

One caregiver in our community once talked about what she called the "many last times." These included:

- The last time she had a meaningful conversation with her husband.
- The last time he helped her with a project around the house.
- The last time she felt comfortable leaving him alone so she could get some time to herself.
- The last vacation they took together.
- The last time he drove.
- The last time he remembered her birthday.

The last times keep coming. The heartbreaks keep coming.

And when our loved ones with dementia pass away, that's when the "many first times" start to pile up.

The first time you mark the widow box on an official form. The first time you celebrate your anniversary without them.

The first time someone asks how your loved one is doing and you have to tell them they have passed away. The first time they aren't there for the holidays.

The first time you call out their name or search for them only to realize they are no longer there.

There is no clean ending to this kind of grief. It arrives in waves. Sometimes the water is calm. Sometimes it crashes without warning. But it doesn't go away.

Trying to avoid these feelings or outrun them is like trying to stop the waves. It will exhaust you, and it will not work.

Most people recognize the grief of watching someone they love change. Watching abilities fade. Watching pride dissolve. Watching others pull away. Watching someone you love become okay wearing the same clothes for days when they once took such care in their appearance.

But there is another grief that often goes unnamed.

The grief of canceled invitations.

The grief of no longer receiving invitations at all.

The grief of losing your partner as your support system, even though they are still physically here.

The grief of handling finances, repairs, and decisions that used to be shared.

The grief of realizing your life is on hold while others move forward.

Caregivers have shared words like these with me:

"I feel like I'm no longer a person, just a caregiver."

"I have to keep smiling and bury the hurt."

"I don't recognize myself anymore."

"I'm suffering in silence."

"I don't need more sympathy. I need help."

There is so much grief in dementia caregiving. And because of that, it makes sense that caregivers don't feel happy or okay all the time. The idea that you should feel positive, grateful, or strong at every stage often adds another layer of pain.

After one of my keynote presentations, a man caring for his wife with Alzheimer's disease came up to me. He looked exhausted and heartbroken. He asked, "What can I do to stop feeling so heartbroken?"

I told him something I believe deeply: "Your heartbreak is a sign of your love. If you did not love her so much, it would not hurt this much."

This grief is not something to fix or rush through. It is something to acknowledge. To make room for. To understand as part of this journey.

You are not weak for feeling it.

You are human.

Chapter 17

Things That Don't Make You a Bad Caregiver

I hope this chapter helps you release the quiet shame about thoughts and moments that are actually common responses to prolonged strain.

I've met some of the most devoted, attentive, loving caregivers in the world.

People who show up every day, who sacrifice deeply, who care more than they ever imagined they could.

And they still have thoughts like:

- *"I don't like my loved one anymore."*
- *"Sometimes I can't stand him."*
- *"I resent her."*
- *"I wish this were over."*

These thoughts don't make them bad caregivers.

They make them human.

More than that, when caregivers name these thoughts out loud, something important happens. The room gets quieter. Other people breathe a little easier. Someone else thinks, *Oh. I'm not the only one.*

If you're having negative thoughts about someone you love, it doesn't mean there's something wrong with you. It usually means you're carrying more than one human nervous system was meant to hold.

Thoughts like these are not plans. They are not wishes. And they are *not* a reflection of how much you love your person.

They are often the mind's way of releasing pressure when the weight gets too heavy. When there is no space to rest, no room to be angry, and no permission to say, *this is more than I can hold*, the mind looks for an outlet.

You can love someone deeply and still feel resentment toward them.

Having a thought does not mean you agree with it. It does not mean you want it to be true. And it does not mean you are failing at caregiving. It means your system is under strain.

And it doesn't stop at thoughts.

Some of the most loving caregivers I've met have, at times, let a loved one sit in stained clothing longer than they would have liked.

They've ignored a question being asked for the fifteenth time that day.

They served cereal for dinner because that was all the energy they had left in that moment.

These moments are not signs of neglect or a lack of love.

They are signs of limited capacity. Of nervous systems stretched thin. Of people doing the best they can with what they have left.

Many caregivers worry about how these moments look from the outside. A stranger sees cereal for dinner. A visitor notices stained clothing. What they don't see are the hours before, the nights without sleep, the behaviors you're managing, or the decisions you've already made that day. A single snapshot during a difficult moment is not the whole story, and you don't have to spend your energy explaining yourself to someone who only sees snapshots.

This isn't personal. It isn't a character flaw or a caregiving failure. It's a reflection of how human nervous systems work. When we are under sustained stress, sleep-deprived, emotionally overloaded, and carrying more responsibility than one person was ever meant to hold, we function in survival mode rather than thriving mode. It's a built-in safety response that allows us to keep going.

This is not permission to neglect a loved one. It's an acknowledgment of what caregiving actually looks like for many people, and that reality is nothing to be ashamed of.

You are not reading this book because you don't care. It's because you care a lot. Enough to replay moments. Enough to wonder whether you should be doing more, or doing it differently. Caring this deeply changes how you think, how you feel, and how you move through the day, often in ways you never anticipated.

Caregiving does not draw from a limitless supply of effort. It draws from capacity. And capacity changes with stress, sleep, health, and emotional load.

On some days, there is room to be patient, creative, and responsive. On other days, there is only enough energy to get through the essentials. That's a normal part of being human, and not something you need to judge yourself for.

Chapter 18

Judgment Has No Place Here

I recently met someone new. When she found out what I do, she responded the way many people do. She told me about a family member with dementia. She shared stories about her grandfather and how his needs eventually increased.

Then she said something in passing, as if it were a universal truth. "Of course, we cared for him at home."

Of course.

That phrase stuck with me.

I know she meant well. I know it came from love.

Most people don't mean harm when they say things like this. Often, they're repeating ideas they've absorbed without realizing how complex caregiving decisions really are.

But underneath comments like that is an assumption many caregivers carry the weight of: that caring for someone at home is the "right" thing to do, and that anything else somehow falls short.

The reality is far more complicated.

When caregiving is already heavy, judgment often becomes a way people try to make sense of the strain. Sometimes it turns inward, as self-criticism. Sometimes it turns outward, as quiet comparisons or assumptions about what others "should" be doing. Both are understandable responses to pressure, not reflections of who we are at our best.

Not everyone is in the same situation. Not everyone has the same health, the same resources, the same support, or the same behaviors to manage. Not everyone has family members who can help. And not every person with dementia has needs that can safely be met at home.

If you want to care for your loved one at home, that can be a beautiful and meaningful choice.

If you decide that a care facility or additional support is the best option, that can be a loving and responsible choice, too.

What's difficult is how quickly judgment creeps in from the outside, often from people who haven't had to live inside these decisions.

I have been in homes where caregivers are pushed far beyond what most people could imagine. I have worked with caregivers who are isolated, exhausted, and quietly afraid. And I have seen situations that make the idea of "of course" fall apart entirely.

I once worked with an elderly woman whose husband had dementia. While I was speaking with her, he walked up and began choking her.

In moments like that, many caregivers feel pressure to tolerate situations that are no longer safe, confusing self-sacrifice with love.

These aren't theoretical questions. They are real decisions caregivers face, often without guidance and often under the weight of other people's expectations and judgments.

There is no single "right" way to care for someone with dementia.

There is only what is safest, most humane, and most sustainable for everyone involved.

Judgment ignores context. It ignores risk. It ignores the invisible toll caregiving takes over time. And it ignores the fact that dementia is not static. Needs change. Behaviors change. What was possible last year may no longer be possible today.

If we could step into each other's homes, witness the sleepless nights, the fear, the impossible choices, and the quiet grief, we would be far less quick to judge.

Caring in Action: Caregiving decisions are not moral tests. They are responses to complex, deeply personal realities. What is right for you may not be right for someone else. And that does not make either choice wrong.

Remember:

- You do not owe anyone proof of your devotion.
- You owe yourself and your loved one safety, care, and compassion.

And sometimes, the most loving decision is the one that others will never fully understand.

Chapter 19

Feelings No One Warned You About

"I thought it was just me."

There are parts of dementia **caregiving** that are painful but expected. The exhaustion. The grief. The frustration.

And then there are experiences that catch you off guard.

Feelings that don't get talked about often.

Thoughts that feel uncomfortable to admit, even to yourself.

This chapter is about naming some of those moments.

Guilt When You Feel Okay

Sometimes, a wave of guilt shows up when you catch yourself actually enjoying something.

A quiet afternoon.

A laugh with a friend.

A few hours where dementia is not front and center.

It can feel almost wrong to feel okay when your loved one is struggling.

As if by experiencing joy, you are somehow taking something away from them. As if your relief means their suffering matters less.

It doesn't.

There is no amount of joy you can withhold from yourself that will change your loved one's dementia. There is no amount of suffering you can take on that will make this disease kinder.

And yet, guilt is incredibly common.

Usually it comes from thoughts like:

- *I shouldn't be doing this.*
- *I should be there.*
- *It's not fair that I get a break and they don't.*

Guilt is a feeling, which means it comes from a thought.

And underneath that thought is almost always the same message.

I've done something wrong.

But when I ask caregivers to slow down and look at the facts, that belief rarely holds up.

Taking a break.

Accepting help.

Making a decision your loved one doesn't like but that keeps them safe.

Those are not moral failures.

They are realities of caregiving.

What's often happening is not that you've done something wrong.

It's that your mind is running an old habit loop that no longer serves you.

Hiding Your Joy

When I was caring for my dad, there were times I felt ashamed to take time for myself.

I remember going up to my cabin for a short break. A quiet place surrounded by pine trees, cooler air, and a little space to breathe. And yet, instead of fully resting, I noticed a strange thought.

I didn't want my siblings to know.

Somewhere in my mind was the belief that if they knew I could get away, maybe they would think my dad wasn't really that bad. Maybe they would think I was exaggerating how much help he needed. Maybe it would make what I was carrying feel smaller in their eyes.

There was another layer, too.

I felt guilty enjoying anything while my dad was miserable. He hated where he was living. He was angry. He was unhappy. And part of me felt like I should be unhappy, too.

So there I was, in a peaceful place, while my mind was at war.

Not because rest was wrong.

But because guilt followed me there.

Looking back, what stands out most is this:

- When my dad died, no one mentioned the times I went to the cabin.
- No one mentioned the help I hired.
- No one tallied the moments I rested versus the moments I sacrificed.
- And no one showed up with a prize.

That realization matters.

Because many caregivers live as if there's a finish line where sacrifice is rewarded.

As if doing everything alone earns special recognition.

It doesn't.

Caregiving is hard no matter how you do it.

With help or without.

With rest or without.

With kindness toward yourself or with constant self-criticism.

If it's going to be hard either way, choose the version that gives you some relief.

Let Others Contribute to Care

Many caregivers tell me they avoid asking for help because they don't want to be a burden. I understand that instinct deeply.

But once, a member of my community pulled me aside and said something that stuck with me. She told me that she and others wanted to help. That they could see how much I was carrying.

And when I explained that I did not want to pressure anyone or make them feel obligated, she gently said, "By not letting us help, you're taking away our chance to contribute. We want to feel useful, too."

That was the first time I really saw this from the other side.

Sometimes, accepting help is not about burdening others. It's about giving them the opportunity to show up, to feel valued, to contribute in a way that matters to them.

Refusing help may protect others from discomfort in the moment.

But it almost always guarantees more discomfort for you.

And again, there is no prize for doing this alone.

When Your Emergency Contacts Disappear

One Careblazer once said something that stopped me in my tracks. "My emergency contacts are disappearing."

She was talking about the quiet realization that the person she once relied on in a crisis could no longer help her.

She told me about a vacation where she fell and severely injured her back. Her husband, who had dementia, saw her fall. Saw her in pain. Saw her lying on the floor. And then went back to watching television, unable to understand what was happening.

She eventually needed back surgery.

At that moment, she realized that the person who once would have helped her through an emergency could not do so anymore.

This is a kind of loss that is rarely acknowledged.

You may not be alone physically. But you start to feel incredibly alone emotionally.

You're alone in a way that is hard to explain.

You may feel like a widow even though your spouse is still alive.

You may feel unsupported even while caring for someone full time.

Because many caregivers think they are weak for feeling this way.

They are not.

They are grieving something very real.

Care in Action: There is no amount of sacrifice that will cure dementia.

There is no version of caregiving where giving more makes this disease fair.

So let's stop glorifying unnecessary suffering.

Let's stop confusing self-denial with love.

Let's stop judging ourselves and each other.

Accepting help.

Taking breaks.

Allowing yourself moments of relief.

These are not betrayals.

They are how caregivers survive.

Afterword

Most books end with a sense of resolution.

A lesson learned.

A problem solved.

A clear ending.

Dementia doesn't work that way.

There is no tidy conclusion. No moment where everything makes sense again. No chapter where the disease stops changing the rules. In that sense, this book doesn't have a happy ending.

It has a heartbreaking one.

And I don't say that to discourage you. I say it because it's true. And because pretending otherwise often makes caregivers feel more alone, not more hopeful.

Dementia caregiving is a journey filled with loss, adjustment, and constant changes. Just when you feel like you've found your footing, something shifts. A new behavior appears. A familiar strategy stops working. Another piece of the person you love quietly slips away.

That does not mean you failed.

It means the disease kept going.

This book was never meant to fix dementia.

It was meant to help you make sense of what is happening, and to suffer less inside it.

There is no happy ending to work toward.

There is only this moment, and the next one, and how you choose to meet them.

And still, many caregivers discover something they did not expect.

A deeper trust in yourself.

A strength you never asked for but now carry.

A knowing that you are capable of more than you ever imagined.

If you take nothing else from these pages, I hope you take this:

You were never meant to do this perfectly.

You were never meant to do this alone.

And you were never meant to do this without it hurting.

The goal of dementia caregiving is not mastery. It is not constant calm. It is not getting every response "right."

The goal is to reduce unnecessary suffering where you can, respond in ways that don't make things harder, and protect yourself so you can keep going.

Some days, that will look like patience and grace.

Other days, it will look like survival and exhaustion.

Both count.

You may not always feel strong.

You may not always feel hopeful.

You may not always like the version of yourself that shows up.

That does not mean you are doing this wrong.

If this book helped you reframe even one difficult moment, soften one interaction, or release one layer of self-blame, then it has done its job. You do not need to apply every strategy. You do not need to remember every chapter. You can return to these pages as often or as little as you need.

Dementia caregiving isn't about arriving somewhere better.

It's about helping someone who needs you without hurting yourself in the process.

And you do not have to figure that out on your own.

If you are reading this and thinking, *I need more support than a book can give*, you are right. Books can guide, normalize, and steady us. But caregiving is lived in real time, with real exhaustion, real grief, and real moments that do not wait for the next chapter.

If you want ongoing guidance, community, and practical support, you can find that at www.careblazers.com. Everything there exists for one reason: to make this journey feel less isolating and more survivable.

No one should have to carry this alone.

You are doing something incredibly hard.

You are allowed to ask for help.

You are allowed to rest.

There may not be a happy ending to this story.

But there can still be moments of connection.

Moments of relief.

Moments of meaning.

And moments where you realize you are not as alone as you once felt.

That matters.

And so do you.

Acknowledgments

This book would not exist without the caregivers who trusted me with their stories.

To the Careblazers in my programs and community: thank you for your openness, your honesty, and your willingness to share what this journey truly looks like. Your experiences shaped every page of this book. Your stories made these strategies real. And the way you keep showing up, even when it feels unbearable, continues to teach me what love and courage look like under extraordinary strain.

I am deeply grateful to Ashante Thomas, my editor, who saw something in my work early on and invited me to put these teachings into book form. Your belief in this message helped bring it into the world.

Thank you to Jena Barreca, who is the backbone of Dementia Careblazers. You hold everything together in ways no one else sees. You show up when things fall through, and you do more than most people realize. This work would not exist without you. I truly can't imagine doing this without you by my side.

I'm also thankful to the entire team at Wiley/Jossey-Bass for your guidance, professionalism, and dedication to supporting work that centers caregivers.

I want to acknowledge the many supervisors, mentors, and teachers I have had throughout my career who fostered my love for working with older adults and modeled thoughtful, compassionate clinical care. I am also grateful to the nurses, aides, social workers, physicians, therapists, and care staff I have worked alongside over the years, whose dedication continues to shape how I understand dementia care.

To my parents, whose lives and care shaped me both personally and professionally: caring for you changed me, and it continues to inform the way I understand family, loss, and love.

And to my friends and family who supported me while this work took shape, especially Eric Johnson, thank you for believing in me and in the importance of this work.

Most of all, to every caregiver and every person living with dementia whose experiences are reflected here, thank you. Your honesty and courage made this book possible. I hope these pages give back even a fraction of what your stories have given to me.

About the Author

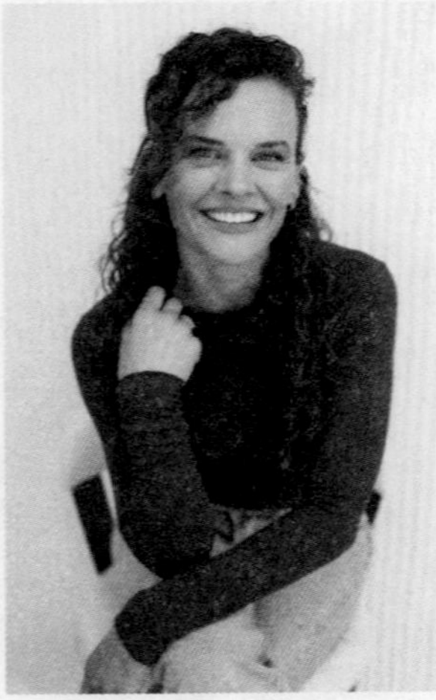

Natali N. Edmonds, PsyD, ABPP (known to many as Dr. Natali), is a dementia care expert, speaker, and consultant who focuses on helping families navigate the emotional and practical realities of caring for a loved one with dementia. She is the founder of Dementia Careblazers, an organization dedicated to supporting family caregivers. A US Army veteran who served in Iraq, Dr. Natali brings a steady, grounded presence to some of life's most overwhelming and uncertain moments.

Through her work, Dr. Natali has reached caregivers across the globe, with more than 28 million views on her educational YouTube channel. She is known for translating complex dementia behaviors into humane, practical responses that reduce guilt, confusion, and burnout. When she is not working with caregivers, she can be found hiking beautiful trails with her rescue dog, Niko, or playing on the pickleball courts. Learn more at www.careblazers.com.

Index

U

W